C000162627

CLIMBING OUT OF A WELL WITH WELLIES ON

**Proof that you can live with
and heal from mental illness**

*A guide to restoring and maintaining mental
wellbeing*

**Kate Birch-Scanlan
BSc(hons) NTDip**

Disclaimer
The information in this book is intended to provide useful information on the subjects discussed. This book is not meant to be used nor should it be used to diagnose or treat any medical condition. Consult your own physician for any diagnosis or medical treatment of a problem.

The publisher and author are not responsible for any specific health or allergy needs that may require supervision and are not liable for any damages or negative consequences that may occur to any person reading or following the information in this book.

References provided are for informal purposes only.

This book is dedicated to Joe and Effie, the two biggest inspirations in my life.

With out knowing it you both have taught me so much and given me the strength to keep going no matter how hard life gets.

Without my life experiences coming together with yours and us having our wonderful chats this book would never have come about.

Special Thanks

Special thanks to Darren Birch-Scanlan for your never-ending patience and proof-reading skills. David Maynard, the best psychotherapist on the planet and the calmest man I've ever met. Dr Robert Davis, my GP who believed me and believed in me. Simon Price, Keith Coupland and Jane McGraham, for your wealth of knowledge and helping me to believe in my abilities and giving me the support to spread my experiences through recovery services and making the idea of this book a reality.

"I came to terms with not fitting in a long time ago. I never really fitted in. I don't want to fit in. And now people are buying into that."

Alexander McQueen

CONTENTS

What it is Like to Live with a Mental Illness

I'm not sure what it's like for you, but for me having a mental illness was like being stuck down a dark well and trying to climb out whilst wearing wellies!

At my worst, I felt I was stuck in this really deep hole, it felt impossible to get out of. Friends, family, colleagues and doctors couldn't hear what I was saying because metaphorically speaking I was too far away from them down the well. It felt like my voice had faded away to nothing by the time it finally reached the top of the well where they were and nothing I said could be heard.

As time moved on, more and more people forgot about me because I didn't mix due to being stuck down the well. Sometimes I'd start to make some headway, begin to see some light. Things would start to move forwards and I was able to climb a little way out of the well only to fall back down again. It was really hard work because I couldn't grip with my feet to climb out due to the wellies I was wearing, and I couldn't take them off.

I'd have moments of real encouragement where I felt like I was making progress, then all of a sudden it would rain, the sides of the well would go slippery and I'd fall back to the bottom again where my voice could no longer be heard.

It was lonely, cold, isolating and frustrating. Every so often a brick would fall down the well from nowhere causing physical pain.

Over time and through making many mistakes I realised that I didn't have to be stuck in the well forever. Although I couldn't remove the wellies, I could create more grips on the soles to enable me to climb out into daylight.

I wrote this book so I could share with others how I climbed out of the well and into the sunlight, in the hope that I could help others reach the sunlight too.

AVOIDING THE TRAP

One trap that people frequently fall into and I did this myself, is waiting for doctors, psychiatrists or psychotherapists to fix things, for medications to take away all symptoms, someone else to wave a magic wand and instantly make everything alright.

I would sit on waiting lists making no progress, usually deteriorating or attend appointments but end up feeling like nothing had changed because I wasn't looking at the bigger picture and neither were the doctors, they were just working on an isolated area.

I had the power to make a difference to my own recovery whilst I waited on lists or attended appointments, I just was not aware of how much I could do to help myself.

The stress and worry of being mentally unwell, the frustration of being stuck on a long waiting list or not seeming to get anywhere within the mental health services is not only distressing for the client but also for their friends and family too. Clients are vulnerable during these times and relapses are common, so the pressure on family and friends can be immense.

Whilst waiting for treatment or working with professionals it is important that you take responsibility for your own wellbeing and continue to work on other areas of your wellbeing outside of that treatment, such as diet, exercise, social interaction, relaxation and sleep because these really matter.

Even though having a mental illness can be very scary, you need to take responsibility for your own recovery. You may not feel like you can do this right now but, believe me given time you will be able to!

By increasing your own knowledge regarding what you can do to help yourself you will gain the strength and power to take onus of your own recovery.

Nobody else is going to make you better, only you can do this. People can guide you, but they can't do it for you.

Introduction

I began writing this book initially to help myself stay on track with my own recovery journey, recovering from both mental and physical illness. After having been diagnosed with a multitude of mental health problems, Fibromyalgia, Myalgic Encephalomyelitis (M.E) and a chronic back problem I was feeling pretty bleak about the future and needed to do something in order to prevent myself from sinking any further and in all honesty to survive.

I'm one of those people who in order to retain information, I need to have everything written down or I'll forget it. Every time I came across something which helped me to feel a bit better, I kept a note, researched it further, sometimes adapted it until eventually I ended up with a set of fourteen steps which helped enable me to improve and maintain my mental health long term.

I focused mainly on my mental health as this indirectly improved my physical health, physical health conditions tend to take their toll on you mentally anyway if they continue for long enough. Although, I did have to work on becoming much more aware of my body and listening to the messages that my body was giving me rather than ignoring them as I used to do.

Mental health support where I live is poor, in fact

mental health care is skeletal now in a majority of areas, but much worse in smaller towns. Waiting lists are exceptionally long and you have to be in a much more distressed and extreme state today to qualify for treatment than you would have to have been several years ago.

Whilst on this journey I came across many people where I live, a small town in Gloucestershire called Tewkesbury, who were unable to get any support towards their own mental health recovery in the same way that I had been struggling to. So, I also began writing this book as a source of support for them as well. Something for them to refer to whilst they were sat on waiting lists, a resource for those with mental health conditions (referred to by the services as clients), carers, parents and friends so that they felt less helpless during some really harrowing, stressful and upsetting times.

You see, Tewkesbury is a reasonably small place in the eyes of the health authorities (it has a population of approximately 20,000) and when it comes to distributing out the money for resources Tewkesbury comes low down on the list of priorities alongside other small towns due to its small population compared to neighbouring towns and cities. Unfortunately, there are a large number of unsupported mental health clients in the community here and unless they know what to look out for and usually pay for, they are often left in a rut to deteriorate.

You would be made to believe by the authorities that

clients have easy access to facilities in neighbouring towns, but this is an unrealistic expectation that has been placed on clients in smaller towns and villages, as many are unable to transport themselves or cope with public transport for the more lengthy journeys.

Years ago, there were more places to attend for support in smaller towns (and larger towns) and transport was provided to help clients get to where they needed to go. Clients made reasonable progress and certainly were not as isolated and depressed as they are now, but due to outsourcing of services and financial cuts this is no longer the case.

To be honest, the real problem is that we are in the midst of a mental health crisis in this country and people are unsupported, placed under too much stress and often don't know how to look after themselves mentally and physically in this increasingly demanding technological and often impersonal world.

Even though we are able to contact people anywhere at any time we are still the loneliest and most depressed that we have ever been. Resources have been stripped back to a bare minimum. Smaller towns like mine have very little facilities and support structure to treat mental health clients with dignity, placing a bigger burden on GP's and the already overstretched larger and more centralised facilities in bigger towns and cities.

Unfortunately, this kind of skeletal setup is never going to cut the mustard when it comes to breaking the back of the enormity of the mental health problems that this country is facing.

We have larger numbers than ever of young people experiencing mental health issues such as self-harm, body dysmorphia, eating disorders, anxiety disorders and depression plus increased numbers of homeless individuals, many with mental health problems. There are abandoned service men and women with little or no psychological support, plus more and more adults experiencing mental health symptoms either for the first time or repeated reoccurrences of pre-existing unsupported conditions.

To add to this, special needs support in schools has also been stripped right back, leading to many children being left with inadequate support or undiagnosed at all. In our case, our children were left unsupported for many years, which resulted in our family being placed under immense pressure and our children experiencing unnecessary symptoms of stress and anxiety, which we had to deal with as a family on top of what turned out to be when finally diagnosed during their teenage years as dyslexia and attention deficit disorder.

Leaving children unsupported in this way is placing a huge extra burden on the already overstretched and undervalued GP's, emergency services, teachers and pastoral care staff who are unable to provide adequate support.

Even with all the available mounting evidence and statistics, still the government doesn't seem to fully acknowledge the link between the need to prioritise providing adequate mental health care and alleviation of stress on other services and resources and how this impacts us as a country.

Although this book cannot replace the missing services and support, it does give you some insight into how you can help support yourself or someone else in a safe way and give you the reassurance that there are still people out there chipping away, trying to create change to the ever decreasing services and also looking out for you even when you feel isolated and alone.

This journey is about making lifestyle changes that will benefit you not only now but throughout your life. To enable you to feel empowered, more resilient and teach you easy skills and tools to help you to cope with tough and stressful periods within your life both with confidence and independently.

Maybe you can even share your newfound knowledge with your friends, family and colleagues too!!

There are fourteen steps in this book which sounds a lot, but really, it's not when you look at them.

I 'm hoping that you will find it manageable to incorporate some or all of these changes into your life gradually over time and eventually maintain them on a daily basis as much as possible. I have included log pages at the back for you to photocopy and fill in to help you to maintain momentum. These will be of particular importance when times are a little more rocky but, are also helpful for maintenance when times are good to maintain both your mental and physical health, improve your resilience to knocks life may throw at you and make your life more enjoyable and fulfilling.

My Journey

Mental illness is something that has always been a part of my life, members of my family have had to carry the burden at certain times of their lives but it also became a serious reality for me when I was 14 years old and became diagnosed with body dysmorphia, depression, anxiety and obsessive compulsive disorder, a black cloud that I carried around with me for many years to come.

My school life was heavily tainted by having to manage the serious symptoms that came along with these conditions, such as obsessive washing, constant checking, anxiety and depression. I was out of school as much as I was in school. In those days nobody really asked you about your mental health unless you were outwardly exhibiting very worrying signs. I managed to get through school achieving A levels in Biology, Chemistry and Physics.

 I went on to Study for an Honours Degree in Biochemistry at the University of Sussex. My time there was tough but there were also some good times, at one point I almost dropped out due to the severity of my condition, but due to the support of my very understanding Sub Dean I didn't and made it to the end.

Following this I went on to secondary school teacher training, but this really was not for me. I think I can safety say after this experience that I am not a 'coping with teenagers on mass' type of person! One or two is fine but thirty, NO!

The world of work followed I got a job creating organic detergents at a local business. I was determined to be 'normal', I had a good degree and wanted a career like anyone else, so I dug my heels in and kept going. Unfortunately, this turned out to be to my own detriment as I ignored and missed the warning signs that were shouting out to me that I was not coping. It wasn't long into my new job that life became too much for me. I was unable to maintain the coping strategies and routines that I had created as a means of getting through each day and I ended up walking away from my job and being placed in a psychiatric hospital to recover.

I never did really gain a lot of benefit from being in hospital, it was just a place where I was overmedicated and sat around smoking, neither of which were of much benefit to my health, but it did give me some space from the pressures of everyday life and I did learn about the lives of some incredibly interesting people and what they'd been through.

After a year, I was eventually allowed to leave hospital and became pregnant with my first child. This was a worrying time, but I adjusted well to motherhood much to everyone's surprise. Eighteen months after the birth of my first child I gave birth to my second child. My second pregnancy really took its toll on my body. It revealed that I had a long term painful back injury from years of sport as a child and it was also during this time that I began experiencing symptoms of Fibromyalgia and Myalgic Encephalomyelitis (M.E).

By the time I was 29 years old I was riddled with widespread pain, debilitating fatigue, depression, anxiety and PTSD (post traumatic stress disorder), plus a collection of other mental and physical illness symptoms, far too many to mention.

One day it all became too much, I could barely walk any distance due to the constant pain and fatigue. I was unable to sleep even though I was exhausted, my anxiety levels were through the roof as was my depression and I couldn't care for my family properly. There seemed to be nothing that the doctors could do to make life any easier. It was easily the worst time of my entire life, I wanted it all to end, I wanted to end it all.

I went to the local hospital in a real mess. I was offered even more pain killers, morphine and lithium, but I was really reluctant to take anything else. I felt it would make me even less able to function, not that there is any shame in anyway in taking medication and I know many people who do successfully, but on this occasion I didn't feel that more medication was the right choice for me. It was at this point that I said to myself there must be something more that I can do to help myself.

The mental health services did not exist where I lived to support me anymore and the doctors had exhausted many of the pharmaceutical options.

The one thing that I had to my advantage was my biochemical knowledge. It was an area that I thought had become a distant memory, but I began to see that it was my way out.

I began looking at my life through a scientist's eyes and I was the subject of my own research. I could see that there were certain aspects of the way that I was living my life that were exacerbating my conditions. One of the areas which I quickly realised I had an influence over, and which others could step in and support me with was my diet.

My diet was pretty poor at this time, made up of lots of convenience and processed foods. These types of foods I felt were potentially contributing to inflammation in my body and this inflammation was then having an effect on my pain and mental health symptoms. So, I set out on a journey to identify foods that helped, foods that maybe exacerbated my conditions and researched how diet could be used to potentially stabilize and improve my health alongside other methods.

Dietary change was not however the answer on its own, although it did make a massive difference. I also had to work on the way I was thinking, how I reacted to situations, my fitness levels and my quality of sleep.

This may sound a lot, but please don't panic just yet! It was not as difficult as it initially appeared it might be when I broke it down into small steps like the ones laid out in this book.

Recovery from and management of a mental illness is made up of many different aspects and varies considerably from person to person. This book is aimed to be a guide to aid recovery rather than strict rules to live by.

I much prefer a relaxed and malleable approach to recovery where you pick and choose what works for you and I think it would be helpful if you saw my fourteen steps like sweets in a pick and mix sweet shop where you pick the ones that you like and create a bag of sweets that suits you. Some people will pick all of the sweets and other people only some of them.

The steps that I have built are based upon my scientific knowledge, personal experiences, and the experiences of others. I find it helpful to have methods to try out that have been tested by someone who has experience within mental health and experiences mental illness symptoms.

I have outlined the steps that I took throughout an average day to help me get back on my feet.

Each of the steps is simple but, combined together they produce very powerful effects. The hardest part is committing to doing them regularly and that effort must come from you.

I wanted my life back with my family, I could not take on time consuming self-care activities as I had limited energy and concentration, any lengthy activity would take away much of the precious time and energy that I had and leave me with no time or energy to do what I really wanted to do. I needed to make small achievable adjustments that I could stick to long term as a lifestyle change rather than a quick fix.

After a while of researching and experimenting with my diet I topped up my knowledge further by studying for a diploma in nutritional therapy, I also studied to become an energy therapist. This taught me the importance of paying attention to the energy system within the body and that not everything with recovery is black and white.

Small Changes Add Up

Small changes needed to be made to my lifestyle to undo some of the damage that modern life was doing to my mental health. Modern life is great in many ways but one big way in which it makes us suffer is that it causes us to have our minds always switched on, we are always on high alert. We can be contacted easily at any time of the day or night via our phones and it has become the norm for us to feel stressed and be constantly busy.

Through not having any time to stop and pause to allow my body and in particular my mind to calm down, even for short periods during the day, I was ignoring and missing all the warning signs that things were going wrong within me.

When you are unaware that things are going wrong in your body and mind because of an inability to slow down you are unable to put steps in place to put things right and this makes you susceptible to mental ill health.

The steps one to fourteen take you through the period of one day, showing you changes that can be made to normal everyday activities that we all do automatically as part of our daily routines, to help us live with and recover from mental illness.

I never thought that I would find anything that would help to relieve my symptoms as they were so severe and I'm sure that there are many people out there thinking the exact same thing. What I hope you realise from reading my book is that you are not alone, that although everyone's journey is very different there are things that can be done to either stabilise or improve matters and you can regain your life again.

"I believe depression is legitimate. But I also believe that if you don't exercise, eat nutritious food, get sunlight, get enough sleep, consume positive material, surround yourself with support, then you aren't giving yourself a fighting chance".

Jim Carrey

CHAPTER ONE
Managing Mornings

Mornings can be Hard!

Mornings can be a challenging time, sometimes impossible, especially if you suffer from anxiety and depression or are going through a stressful period such as sitting exams, relationship and family problems, challenges at work, health problems or money worries.

Very often during these times you wake up feeling unrefreshed and exhausted because you have had interrupted sleep. You may have niggling aches and pains in your body which can start to worry you.

Sometimes, you may have a feeling of huge pressure on your shoulders running up into your head giving you a headache, but the worst part often is the anxiety, which you carry around with you each day that never seems to go away.

Something that I have frequently noticed when I have been going through a challenging time (although it can happen for no apparent reason as well) is that I feel anxious over everything! Even the most basic tasks become difficult, sometimes I can't do them at all. There seems to be no rhyme or reason for some of the anxieties that I have, all I can say is that my nervous system is just a lot more sensitive than it used to be due to it being overloaded by the pressures of life and sometimes triggered by past events stored in it.

What happens is my nervous system reacts to every stress or pressure that's occurring as if it's a high-level stress or emergency even when it doesn't need to, resulting in palpitations, worry, exhaustion, butterflies in my stomach and panic attacks. These feelings may sound familiar to many of you.

When you get stuck in an anxiety cycle which is what is described above, whether it's caused by an underlying condition or a stressful event you can over time begin to not feel good enough anymore, you start to doubt your own abilities or question if this situation you are in will ever improve. Your mind and body can go into a 'self-protective' state where it encourages you to hide away in a warm, comfortable place such as your bed, you often feel tired, achy and unmotivated, this is known as sickness behaviour, the type of behaviour noted when we become depressed. Unfortunately, long term this type of behaviour will only make matters worse.

You may be reading this and thinking that this describes where you feel you are at right now or describes someone that you know. Maybe, it has been going on for a while and you wish that you hadn't ignored it, that you wish you had told someone, but you felt a bit daft, a bit of a burden, or if it's someone else you are thinking about that you were interfering. You may have thought by now the feelings would have gone away, but the struggles still continue day in, day out making life really hard. This can make it difficult to work, study, socialise, eat and sleep.

Now, let me reassure you here, all these feelings are very natural and the body's way of trying to help you, even though it doesn't feel like it. In the past these heightened responses were important to you, they enabled humans to escape from predators.

Unfortunately, however, unless you are in immediate danger this level of overreactive nervous system response is no longer beneficial to you and can cause problems to your day to day functioning if you are unable to turn the intensity down. The good news is you can turn this intensity down by making some lifestyle changes.

In many respects, mornings are the most important time of the day. They set the mood for the rest of the day. Something I have found very useful is to work on placing the nervous system in a calmer state very first thing in the morning before anxiety has had chance to fully take hold.

When we are anxious our nervous system is in a constant state of fight or flight, this leaves us feeling hyper alert, exhausted, irritable and unable to cope, plus if we suffer from other mental health conditions it can trigger symptoms of those too.

Having a short nervous system calming routine in the morning can really help us to regain clarity and focus and set us up so we are better able to face the day ahead.

"Our anxiety does not come from thinking about the future, but from wanting to control it."

Kahlil Gibran

If you rearrange the letters in
DEPRESSION

you'll get

I PRESSED ON!

Meaning your current situation is
not your final destination.

Before We Begin!!

Before we begin any of the steps in this book, I just want to bring up something which I feel is important and needs to be highlighted.

This point is **kindness.**

When I say kindness, I'm talking about kindness to one's self.

You will hear time and time again people say to you 'to help yourself you need to be kind to yourself.'

Now, in my experience saying this isn't enough. It doesn't really mean anything to just say 'be kind to yourself.' The driving urge to keep pushing through, the critical voices in your head telling you you're rubbish, fat, ugly, stupid and that you've failed continue to be there.

What I did, which helped me an awful lot to enable me to successfully make changes, was to take a step back and look at myself from the outside, as if looking in as a third person.

I asked myself a few questions:

If I were talking to a friend would I speak to them in the same way that I speak to myself?

How can I heal if the information I feed myself is negative and putting myself down?

What would help some one to grow and heal, encouragement, support, kindness and patience or stern words, punishments and negative self-talk?

If I were able to communicate with the child part of me (a part we all have and which may have been traumatised at some point in the past) and they were to make a mistake and they were punished for it or spoken to negatively, how would they feel in the future, would they become anxious the next time they attempted it?

If your child part were to see making mistakes as a learning curve and they felt supported through this and that it was something that was helping them to grow, would this enable them to approach life with less anxiety and as a lifelong process of learning which can be enjoyable, intriguing, interesting and fulfilling although challenging and painful at times, rather than a time of suffering?

Answering these questions, I'm sure that you will have come to a similar conclusion to me. That in order to feel better we need to be supportive, kind and understanding of ourselves. Accept that sometimes we will feel like we've made mistakes or failed, and this is not a crime, it's just part of the 'normal' flow of life.

Personally, I had to place my mind into a completely different state to what it was used to. This took some work and I would regularly have to bring myself back to what's written on these pages in order not to drift off down a destructive route of self-criticism and punishment and you may have to do a similar thing.

The more you practice bringing your mind back to being supportive and kind to yourself the easier and more natural a process it becomes, and you will begin over time to start treating yourself as a friend rather than an enemy.

Kindness in words creates confidence.

Kindness in thinking creates profoundness.

Kindness in giving creates love.

Lao Tzu

STEP ONE

Calming the Nervous System Before the Day Begins by Breathing into the Heart Area

Breathing exercises which calm the nervous system are as important for the body as eating well, sleeping well, physical exercise and social interaction.

Breathing into the Heart Exercise

Try the following exercise every morning when you wake up.

Each morning when you wake up, lie down or sit on the edge of the bed or on a chair, whichever is most comfortable for you.

Place your hands crossed over your heart area. Feel your body on the bed or your feet on the floor and body on the chair if you are sitting up.

Take a few moments to just focus on your breath, the sensation of it flowing into your body, down to your lungs, the feeling of your abdomen rising and falling and the sensation of the bed, chair or floor beneath you.

Take a deep breath in through your nose. Follow the air flow down to the heart area where your hands are, feel your lungs expand. Don't force the breath. Keep your hands over your heart.

Hold the breath for a moment or two.

Now let the breath go, notice it travel up away from your heart and from your lungs, up through your chest and out through your mouth.

Then on the next breath, breathe into the heart area and then imagine the breath filling your stomach, your legs and the rest of your body right up to your head, pause for a second, then feel it as it flows back to the heart area and out through your mouth again.

Accept any thoughts and feelings that you may have, no need to fight them, just let them be there. When your mind wanders from the breath just gently bring your attention back to the breath.

Repeat this ten times or for as long as you want to.

Future progress:

To progress from this, you could add the phrase 'let go' to this exercise.

So, on the in breath you would say 'let' and on the out breath say 'go'. Feel the tension and worry gently flow out from your body and mind as you breathe out.

Following this if you want to learn more there are good mindfulness meditations on online, plus there are mindfulness courses and meditation classes often run in the community.

One of the greatest gifts that we can give ourselves is to learn how to sit with our thoughts and focus on our breath without feeling like we need to react or change anything about them.

TIP:

You know when you have those times when anxiety keeps bubbling up during the day?

To reduce this breathing exercises, mindfulness and meditations are invaluable tools.

Saved in my phone I have my favourite short meditations always to hand. I would advise you to do something similar yourself, whether it be in your phone or a technique that you store in your mind.

Then during the day whenever things start to stray pause even if just for a couple of minutes and practice your chosen meditation or breathing technique to help bring yourself back into balance.

If you can get into the habit of doing this regularly you are likely to experience less anxiety and mood dips, allowing you to move through life more smoothly.

When you first begin doing this set yourself regular reminders to check in with yourself and to see if your stress levels are building up, because it is unlikely that you will notice the stress mounting if you are used to being on automatic pilot all of the time.

Even now, I give myself a prod from time to time, as my natural reaction is to push through and ignore the signals of stress.

Without Any Counteraction to Some of Our Inbuilt Behaviours We Are Heading Towards Breaking Point

Due to the fact I could not just rely on my own experiences alone, throughout my research for this book I spoke to many different people, young adults, middle aged and older people. I ran recovery groups for a local mental health service and got involved in several mental health organisations. I spent a lot of time talking to amazing people suffering from varying degrees of mental ill health, conditions such as Generalised Anxiety Disorder (GAD), Schizophrenia, Borderline Personality Disorder, Self-harm, Body Dysmorphia, Obsessive Compulsive Disorder, Depression, Anxiety, Bipolar disorder and Eating disorders, plus some with different learning styles such as Dyslexia and Attention Deficit Disorder.

From the lovely people that I spoke to I found that some could sit and do breathing exercises and meditation for 10, 20, 30 minutes, even an hour but many could not and ended up feeling that breathing exercises, relaxation techniques and mediation were just not for them for a variety of different reasons and that they had failed at it.

No one really finds breathing exercises and meditation practices easy at first because often they try to see them as a miracle cure and that's not what their all about. You can't fail when it comes to these kinds of practices, just doing them, whatever the experience you have whilst doing them and the outcome is enough.

When we engage in these practices, it often feels like we are going against how our bodies have been programmed to work.

As we develop from children to adolescents and then adults we are programmed to perform in certain ways, to achieve high grades, be motivated, not rest as it's a sign of weakness, keep going, work long hours, have immaculate homes, exercise to extreme lengths 'No pain, no gain'!!, Without any counteraction or relief from this way of thinking most of us are heading towards breaking at some point.

Breathing exercises and mediations that we are often introduced to in the beginning feel just way too long and uncomfortable. We feel unable to sit with the feelings that we are experiencing at that time in our bodies and minds and this puts us off going down this route.

The whole aim with these exercises is that we begin to be able to sit with these uncomfortable feelings gradually and listen to the feedback our own body is giving us. As this over time allows the feelings the opportunity to settle.

When you are starting out on this journey, if you are anxious or struggle to sit for long, it's better and kinder to start small, such as with the breathing exercise, I have outlined in step one.

Our minds need to rest as much as our bodies, sleep is

very important for this but slowing down our minds and our nervous systems through breathing exercises, mediation and mindfulness are equally as important.

If you have never done much in the way of breathing exercises, then step one is a good place to begin. It is easy and quick to learn and can be used in many different situations to calm you. Even as someone who uses these types of breathing exercises a lot it is an exercise that I continue to use regularly, as I find it effective, especially for anxiety relief and letting go of the pressures of life. It is also an exercise that my children find helpful, as life for them and a vast majority of young people is extremely stressful these days, especially with the pressures now placed on them by schools and social media.

To achieve benefit from these types of practices you only really need to master doing them for short periods of time. The important part is to be consistent and practice every day or at least as often as you can but, ideally every day.

Something that is helpful to do is to identify how the breathing exercises make you feel and to keep a note of your thoughts and feelings after doing the exercises.

Seeing how you felt written down can often help you to stick at them and encourage you to do them again the next day. If you come off track it can help to remind you why you began doing them in the first place.

For example, I wrote:

- It enables me to feel lighter and that I am carrying around less baggage.

- I experience less pain and tension in my body.

- I experience fewer panic attacks.

- My sleep pattern has improved.

- Sometimes difficult feelings come to the forefront, but they tend to cause me less problems afterwards.

Write your experiences in the log section at the back of the book.

ANXIETY

Anxiety is normal part of life, however sometimes it becomes persistent and we need to take steps to reduce it.

Symptoms of anxiety include, increased heart rate, increased muscle tension, tingling hands and feet, breathing too fast, dizziness, feeling sick, hot flushes, headaches, dry mouth, shaking and palpitations.

When you are overly anxious you may think that you are going mad, that you may die, that you are having a heart attack or have a health condition like a brain tumour. You may think that you are going to faint or that people are watching you. Sometimes things may appear to be speeding up or slowing down, you may feel detached from what's around you or have a feeling of wanting to run away.

Even if you are suffering from any of the symptoms above and it feels like a permanent fixture right now, it doesn't have to remain this way, hold on.

CHAPTER TWO

What Are You Grateful for Today?

*"Gratitude" ~ the quality of being thankful, readiness
to show appreciation for and to return kindness.*

Acknowledging what you are grateful for has been
shown through research to increase feelings of
happiness, reduce depression, support our immune
system, help us to feel more alive and sleep better, it
also helps to reduce social comparisons, which during
this time of social media explosion can be effective at
reducing feelings of resentment and reduced self-
esteem.

STEP TWO

Practicing Gratitude

How Can I Practice Gratitude?

Write down or simply just mentally acknowledge 3 things that you are grateful for today. This can be anything at all from having clean water to family, friends, pets or a roof over your head.

1.

2.

3.

Write down how this process made you feel in the log section.

SOCIAL MEDIA

Over the last ten years social media has taken over as a platform for human interaction, but this has come at a cost.

Social media is a big part of our lives and for some an unavoidable part. The amount of evidence for the impact of social media on our mental health is rising.

Social Media Addiction

We've all heard about 'social media addiction'. The addictive nature comes from the urge to check social media usually after posting in order to get a short-term pleasure hit. The pleasure hit occurs as the likes that are received cause dopamine to be released in the brain giving a feeling of instant gratification. The desire for another hit of dopamine causes people to constantly refresh their social media feed.

This is a dangerous road because if gratification is not received the user may believe that they are ugly, unfunny and unpopular, much of these feelings becoming internalised. As a result, the person may post again for personal validation and so the cycle continues.

Sleep

Another area of wellbeing which is impacted is quality of sleep. Studies have shown that using social media compulsively can damage sleep patterns, effecting school or work performance, relationships and general health and wellbeing.

FOMO

The desire to stay connected to what others are doing has generated the concept of 'fear of missing out' FOMO! People fear that they may be missing out on rewarding experiences that others are having and therefore try to stay connected to what others are doing. This can lead to lower mood, reduced life satisfaction, anxiety, loneliness, depression and feelings of inadequacy.

Unrealistic Expectations

The promotion of unrealistic expectations on social media is linked to poor self-esteem and self-image, depression and anxiety. This has been made worse through image manipulation. It gives people, the young in particular, unrealistic expectations of how we should look and behave.

As social media is so dominant within our society, we need to learn how to be able to use it whilst protecting our mental health.

Schools need to start including lessons on this in their timetables and parents should keep an eye on what children have access to, although with teenagers this can be difficult.

Adults need to be sensible about what they post as it's there for any age to see and social media firms need to be making more effort to keep people safe especially from trolling and preventing redirection to inappropriate websites.

As individuals we all need to remember that whatever we post online is going to impact ourselves or someone else.

- *Never post anything about yourself that you are uncomfortable with.*

- *Never say cruel things to others, as the impact on them will be far greater than you imagine, and you could trigger someone to harm themselves.*

- *If negative or cruel things get posted about you remember that this is a reflection of the person posting it, not of you. They are weak, often unhappy or jealous of the life you have and what you have achieved.*

"When I started counting my blessings my whole life turned around".

Willie Nelson

CHAPTER THREE

The Importance of Drinking Enough Water

Do You Drink Enough Water?

Our brains are made up of about 75% water and are dependent on proper hydration to function effectively.

When we don't drink enough water, which many of us don't we can have difficulty concentrating. Dehydration can impair both short-term and long-term memory function. It can also cause headaches, brain fog and changes in mood.

Studies have shown that a loss of water as little as 1.5 percent can alter peoples energy levels and mood.

The longest we go without water is usually during the night which is why it is so important that we drink well when we wake up.

Water is lost from the body through urine, sweat and respiration. We are constantly losing water.

It is recommended that we drink at least 2 litres of water per day.

A red flag for dehydration and that you need to drink more is darker urine!!

STEP THREE

Staying Hydrated

Drink a Glass of Water First Thing in the Morning

First thing in the morning drink a glass of water to rehydrate yourself.

You can add a slice or lemon or lime if you like.

Notice how it makes you feel to drink more water, how it effects your levels of alertness and concentration, your fatigue, any aches and pains and your general mood.

Write your experience of how you feel when you drink more water in the log section.

Continue to regularly tune in with yourself during the day to check that you are not dehydrated. Set an alarm on your phone if it helps. Hydration is very important, but don't go overboard 2-3 litres is plenty and this includes other fluids too, but a large proportion of it being good old plain water is best in my opinion.

Remember you also rehydrate when you eat fruits and vegetables. Watermelon is particularly good.

TIP:

Fill a couple of bottles of water to drink throughout the day. Begin to get into the mindset of staying well hydrated.

She warned him not to be deceived by appearances, for beauty is found from within.

Beauty and the Beast

CHAPTER FOUR

Nutrition and Mental Wellbeing

(Basically, what I wish I had been taught in school!)

Before we even enter into this chapter, and its subsequent steps, I want to make it very clear that this is not a weight loss plan or faddy diet. It doesn't matter if you are fat, thin or somewhere in between. Improvements in health can occur irrespective of weight. Weight loss or weight gain may come as a result of any adjustments that you make depending on where your at, but this is not the focus. I do not believe that weight and our diet should ever be the focus, and nor should it make us feel guilty or miserable.

However, what I am passionate about and feel has been lost within our society is an understanding of how nutritious foods are essential to our mental wellbeing and I believe that it is important that we know why.

You may feel that weight is the cause of your anxiety, social isolation and depression, which it could well be, but focusing on it isn't going to improve matters, learning how to look after yourself and appreciating your body for what it does for you is what counts.

"Beauty begins the moment you decide to be yourself."

Coco Chanel

"Is 'fat' really the worst thing a human can be? Is 'fat' worse than 'vindictive', 'jealous', 'shallow', 'vain', 'boring', or 'cruel'? Not to me."

J K Rowling

If your concentration is poor at this time come back to read this chapter later and move on to step 4.

So, let's begin.

We need to know why basic nutrients are required so we can make informed decisions regarding what we eat. I've met so many people who just have not been taught how nutrition keeps our brains functioning the best that they can.

Eating well and eating regularly are important when it comes to managing and sometimes preventing symptoms of stress, anxiety and depression. It's not as difficult to learn about as you may think.

Personally, I had felt overwhelmed by the nutritional information available particularly online and all the middle-classed cookery books out there made me feel like I was constantly failing.

Due to my scientific background I knew that what I ate would have an impact on how I felt but managing to change my diet was a whole different matter, especially when I felt so ill.

From the journey that I have been on and from helping and observing others, I believe that if people knew why certain nutrients were important to how the body and brain functions, they would be better placed to be positively involved in their own internal dialogue around food particularly during times of difficulty and make food choices which promote and support mental wellbeing.

So, say for example that an individual didn't want to eat because they felt low, anxious or depressed and hadn't eaten for a while, they would know that by eating regularly and consuming nutritious foods and foods containing particular nutrients that their chances of reducing their symptoms was greatly increased, therefore placing them in a more powerful position.

The Gut Brain Axis

Between our gut and our brain there is constant communication. This two-way communication is known as the gut-brain axis. Bacteria in our gut are involved in this communication and it has been shown that by making simple dietary changes we can modify our gut bacteria in such a way as to help symptoms of depression and anxiety.

In the western world we tend to eat a lot of processed foods, refined sugars, fried foods, high fat meats and artificial sweeteners. We also eat lower amounts of fruits, vegetables, whole grains, healthy fats, fish, nuts and seeds which has a negative effect on the state of our digestive system and our mental health. I will talk more about this throughout this chapter.

For anyone experiencing anxiety, in the beginning they just want to feel calmer in order to be able to tackle life's challenges. One important point that we need to remember if we want to feel calmer is that we need to avoid blood sugar peaks and crashes throughout the day. They frequently happen mid-morning or mid-afternoon. Often when we feel low, sugar is one of the first things that we reach for to give us an instant mood boost. However, dips in blood sugar level often occur after we've eaten meals such as sugary cereals for breakfast, chocolate bars, cakes, biscuits, crisps and other refined carbohydrates.

When we eat foods such as these we instantly get a boost in blood sugar which then initiates the production of insulin to enable our cells to take up the sugar that we have eaten, as a result our blood sugar levels drop and we can be left feeling irritable, stressed, with brain fog and craving more of this type of food to give us another mood boost.

Eating foods containing complex carbohydrates in the form of foods such as wholemeal bread, oats, brown rice and vegetables and also consuming protein helps to prevent these blood sugar peaks and troughs.

The meals that I am going to show you in this book are in no way meant to be a regimented diet plan, they are just examples for you to pick and choose from and to later on adapt as you begin to get a feel for what you can do to feel healthier. They are simply just a place to start from. I soon realised on my own journey that so many people just don't know where to begin. As you will see I've paid careful attention to including nutrients which have been scientifically shown to benefit mental wellbeing.

What we are aiming for are small changes in lifestyle that are intended for the long term. They are aimed at balance rather than restriction, it's not a short-term diet with rules to stick to, therefore you cannot fail because there is nothing to fail at.

Another thing to mention is that hopefully you will not find the food mentioned is too expensive and that you are able to work it within your budget. So much advice these days is based on you having enough money to buy the latest fashionable food fad and many people simply don't have that luxury and to be honest it's not necessary anyway.

There Are No 'Good' or 'Bad' Foods

Food is food.

It provides us with nutrients, comfort, pleasure, and connection to others.

It is a wonderful thing.

There are no good, bad, healthy or unhealthy food labels in this book. Labelling them in this way can be damaging to the way that we talk to ourselves and others regarding food. I am simply going to show you which foods are 'more nutritious' and beneficial to our wellbeing and which are less nutritious and may exacerbate symptoms.

It is important to remember that anxiety, depression, stress and other symptoms of mental ill health can be caused and exacerbated by many different triggers therefore, nutrition is only part of the cause and of the solution.

However, nutrition can be a very effective management tool once we know what we are doing and have a little knowledge on the subject. As I say in the heading, I really feel that this should be taught in schools as we all need to eat, and we all experience stressful situations in our lives. Worryingly increasing numbers of children today are suffering from the symptoms of mental health conditions and are not educated in some of the ways they can look after themselves.

Helping yourself through self-care methods such as diet can be very empowering as it's a way that people can actively engage in their own healthcare which is vital for wellbeing and recovery.

You have brains in your head.

You have feet in your shoes.

You can steer yourself any direction you choose.

Dr Seuss

What Is Food Made up of?

The composition of food is categorised into **macro-nutrients** and **micro-nutrients.**

Macro nutrients are the main nutrients that make up the food that we eat. They are required in relatively large quantities.

The main macro-nutrients include:

Carbohydrates (and dietary fibre)

Fats (lipids)

Protein

Carbohydrates

These are the bodies preferred choice of fuel. *They contain carbon, hydrogen and oxygen atoms.*

They can be split into:

Sugars - These are short chain carbohydrates, for example glucose, galactose, fructose and sucrose.

Starches - Which are long chains of glucose molecules that eventually get broken down to glucose by the digestive system.

Nutritious sources of carbohydrates include:

Whole grains such as brown rice, pure oats and quinoa

Beans and lentils

Vegetables

Whole fruit

Less nutritious sources include:

Sugary drinks

Fruit juices

Pastries

White bread

White pasta

White rice

Cakes

Fibre – Dietary fibre keeps everything in the gut moving. When combined with water fibre swells up and triggers contractions in the gut called peristalsis which squeezes everything along in the gut. Bacteria in the digestive system break down fibre, the products of which help maintain the health of the gut lining.

A healthy gut lining is important for both physical and mental wellbeing.

Nutritious sources of fibre include:

Fresh fruit

Fresh vegetables

Whole grains

Beans

Pulses

CARBOHYDRATES

Carbohydrates provide fuel for the nervous system and energy for muscles. They act as a quick energy source and they are important for the brain to function. Eating complex carbohydrates such as beans, peas, lentils, vegetables, wholegrain breads and cereals over simple carbohydrates found in biscuits, cakes and other processed foods provides a steady source of energy helping to avoid blood sugar peaks which do not help our mental health.

Fats

The word 'fat' is often seen as a negative one but not all fats are bad for you. Some fats are vital for mental and physical wellbeing.

Certain fats help to reduce inflammation therefore protecting the body from many health conditions.

Fats are involved in a number of different functions in the body including the absorption of vitamins A, D and E. They are involved in hormone production and they are components of cell membranes. Fats also protect organs within the body and are a great source of energy as they can be stored in the body in times of excess.

Certain fats provide the body with what are known as essential fatty acids, 'essential' meaning that the body cannot make them itself or function without them such as omega 3 and omega 6. Omega 3 fatty acids are found in oily fish and omega 6 fatty acids are found in vegetable oils, eggs, nuts and whole grains. Omega 3 fatty acids are particularly important for mental health.

What Happens When Fats are Broken Down?

When they are needed fats are broken down into glycerol and fatty acids to produce fuel for the body. The glycerol is converted to glucose by the liver and the fatty acids are broken down by a process called beta oxidation. The brain requires certain fatty acids to enable it to function well. Omega 3 is believed to reduce inflammation by counteracting the actions of pro-inflammatory cytokines (cytokines are signalling proteins that are involved in immunity and inflammation) and therefore lessening symptoms of depression. Increased inflammation has been shown in depressed patients.

There are many words used in place of the term fats, such as triglycerides, oils and lipids. In food the main types of fat that we need to be aware of are saturated, unsaturated (monounsaturated and polyunsaturated) and trans fats.

Saturated fats are usually solid and found in foods such as:

Butter

Cheese

Meat

Coconut oil

Palm oil

Unsaturated fats are often liquid and divided into monounsaturated and polyunsaturated, for example:

Monounsaturated:

Olive oil

Avocados

Rapeseed oil

Nuts and seeds

Polyunsaturated:

Omega 3 - Oily fish such as mackerel or salmon

Walnuts

Flaxseed

Omega 6- Sunflower oil

Soya bean oil

Palm oil

Linseed oil

Pumpkin seeds

Poultry

Eggs

Wholemeal bread

Most vegetable oils

Trans fats

There are two forms of trans fats, natural and artificial. The fats which are less nutritious and best eaten in very small amounts are artificial trans fats.

Artificial trans fats are created artificially through a process called hydrogenation. Unfortunately, they can cause a reduction in the levels of good (HDL) cholesterol in the body and increase levels of bad (LDL) cholesterol. They also can cause weight gain and increase risk of heart disease.

Artificial trans fats are found in foods such as:

Cakes

Biscuits

Margarine

Pastries

Fried foods

Natural trans fats occur in meat and dairy products from cattle, sheep and goats. You do not need to overly worry about these fats too much, just consume them in moderation.

OMEGA 3

Omega 3 fatty acids are polyunsaturated fats naturally occurring in fish.

A diet rich in Omega 3 is beneficial as it can boost the number of bifidobacteria in the gut microbiome.

Bifidobacteria are beneficial because they help to digest dietary fibre, prevent infection and produce vitamins.

They help to dampen down inflammation in the body which is believed to be connected to reducing symptoms of depression and anxiety.

Mackerel, salmon, herring and sardines contain high levels of omega 3.

Nutritious sources of fats include:

- Oily fish
- Olive oil
- Avocados
- Eggs
- Nuts
- Seeds
- Olives

Less nutritious sources of fats include:

- Margarine
- Corn oil
- Biscuits
- Cakes
- Crisps
- Fried foods
- Anything containing hydrogenated vegetable oil

Proteins

Proteins are made up from many units called amino acids all joined together.

Most animal protein sources are 'complete' proteins which means that they contain all the 9 amino acids that the body needs to function, but not many plant sources are complete protein sources.

Quinoa, buckwheat and soya are complete plant protein sources. Vegetarians and vegans often need to combine plant sources to create a meal complete in protein.

Protein is required for building muscle, but also some amino acids from protein are the precursors for certain neurotransmitters in the body which are important for mental health such as dopamine and serotonin.

Dopamine regulates movement, attention, learning and emotional responses. It is involved in the reward centre in the brain.

Dopamine plays a role in addiction and is central to our motivation. When our dopamine levels are low, we can feel fatigued, demotivated, sad, hopeless, anxious, have mood swings, low energy, be unable to focus, have stiff, aching muscles and disturbed sleep. But when dopamine levels are adequate, we experience more pleasure and satisfaction and are better able to keep our attention and regulate our emotions.

Serotonin, often called the happy hormone regulates anxiety, happiness and mood. Low levels of serotonin are associated with depression.

Nutritious sources of protein include:

Meat

Fish

Eggs

Dairy products

Nuts

Seeds

Beans

Lentils

PROTEIN

When we eat proteins, they are broken down into amino acids, which are the bodies building blocks for growth and energy.

The amino acid tryptophan is used in the synthesis of serotonin, this is the hormone which reduces symptoms of depression and anxiety.

Unprocessed animal protein sources such as meat, poultry, fish and eggs provide your body with all the amino acids that your body needs. Plant based proteins such as grains, beans, vegetables and nuts often lack one or more essential amino acids, so you may need to eat a combination of them to get all the amino acids that you need for your brain to function well.

Fibre

Some people call fibre 'roughage' This is the part of plant foods that we are unable to digest. It is a type of carbohydrate that keeps our digestive system healthy. Fibre can be either soluble or insoluble.

Bacteria in the digestive system break down fibre producing a substance called butyrate which helps control the growth of cells lining the gut but also has powerful anti-inflammatory effects.

Soluble fibre is prebiotic, which means it feeds bacteria in our gut improving our gut microbiome. Our gut microbiome is the ecosystem of different organisms that live in our gut such as bacteria, yeasts, fungi and viruses. An imbalance of our gut bacteria has been connected to anxiety, depression and inflammation in the body. It is an area which is actively being researched as a treatment for depression and anxiety which has shown some promising results.

It is important that we pay attention to building up populations of beneficial gut bacteria in our gut.

We can increase the populations of beneficial gut bacteria by:

- Eating a diet high in fruit and vegetables and as diverse as possible.

- Including fermented foods like sauerkraut, kefir and kimchi.

- Eating prebiotic foods such as mushrooms, as they feed the 'good' gut bacteria.

- Including resistant starch, for example beans, peas and lentils, oats, cooled and reheated potatoes and pasta.

  Resistant starch is a form of starch that can't be digested by the small intestine and is fermented by bacteria in the large intestine producing short chain fatty acids such as butyrate which are used as a source of energy for the cells in the colon, improving the health of the cells in the gut and preventing abnormal cell formation.

- Getting outside more, exercising, opening your windows, avoiding unnecessary antibiotics, owning a dog and gardening also help to support our gut microbiome.

Insoluble fibre either acts as a bulking agent enabling us to remove waste from the body or as a prebiotic feeding the bacteria in our gut. Another reason why it is important is because it's involved in a number of functions such as reducing cholesterol, lowering the pH of the gut to increase absorption of minerals and stimulating various immune cells.

Eating enough fibre is linked to decreased risk of many health conditions including reduced risk of diabetes and bowel cancer. It's recommended that we aim for around 30g per day for adults.

Sources of soluble fibre include:

Oats

Black and kidney beans

Brussel sprouts

Avocados

Sweet potatoes

Broccoli

Pears

Figs

Apricots

Carrots

Apples

Flaxseeds

Sunflower seeds

Sources of insoluble fibre include:

Wholegrains such as brown rice and couscous

Nuts

Seeds

Fruit and vegetable skins

FIBRE

Scientific understanding of the connection between the gut and the brain has increased over recent years.

Fibre has been shown to be a very beneficial component when it comes to improving gut health and reducing stress.

Research has shown that people eating a diet containing plenty of fibrous foods are likely to experience less stress and anxiety.

The recommended dietary fibre intake for an adult is 30g per day.

Adding some fibrous foods to each meal such as fruits, vegetables, pulses, nuts, seeds, whole grains and oats is the easiest way to increase your fibre intake.

Healing is not linear

Micro-nutrients

Micro-nutrients are vitamins and minerals. They are required by the body in very small amounts.

Vitamins A, E and K are fat soluble and are stored in the liver, for this reason you don't need them every day, but you require them regularly.

Vitamin C and the B vitamins (of which there are several B vitamins) are water soluble and are required every day because they can't be stored by the body.

Minerals are compounds found in most of the foods we consume. They are crucial to basic bodily functions and the range of processes that they help to regulate is nearly endless.

Minerals required by the body include:

Calcium	Iodine
Magnesium	Selenium
Phosphorus	Fluoride
Potassium	Copper
Sodium	Manganese
Chloride	Chromium
Zinc	
Iron	

To remain as well as possible we need to aim to gain nutrients from all food groups, but there are some nutrients which are considered of particular importance when it comes to mental health.

Nutrients that are particularly important for mental health are:

Omega 3

Magnesium

Calcium

Zinc

B vitamins - Especially B12 and B6

Vitamin D - Page 128

Iron

Selenium

Vitamin E

Omega 3

Omega 3 fatty acids are vital for the brain and the nervous system. They are essential for maintaining the structure of the myelin sheath, which is the insulating sleeve of fatty tissue that protects nerve cells allowing signals to flow down the nerve at the right speed.

The myelin sheath which surrounds nerves is constantly breaking down and rebuilding and we need to provide it with the right nutrients to do so. It is made from fats plus a few proteins, the protein part we can assemble ourselves but some of the most important fats need to come from our diet, in particular an omega 3 fatty acid called DHA (docosahexaenoic acid). If we don't eat enough DHA the myelin sheath can become damaged meaning that the nerve cells do not fire properly, and reception of neurotransmitters is affected.

Studies have shown that omega 3 fatty acids can support our nervous system and decrease inflammation. Inflammation has been connected to many health conditions including mental health issues.

There is strong evidence that supplementation with omega 3 can reduce depressive episodes via its anti-inflammatory actions.

Sources of Omega 3:

To obtain the essential long chain omega 3 fatty acids we need to eat oily fish or grazing cattle. You can also take an omega 3 supplement ideally containing 750mg EPA (eicosapentaenoic acid) and 250mg DHA daily but check with your doctor or health professional first.

Vegans struggle to get enough EPA. They are able to get short chain omega 3 fatty acids from flax seeds, chia seeds and walnuts, but to get the essential longer chain fatty acids they need to take an Omega 3 supplement made from Algae which contains both DHA and EPA.

Omega 6

You may also have heard about omega 6. It tends to get bad press, but it is critical to brain function as well. The problem is we tend to eat too many sources of omega 6 and not enough sources of omega 3.

The ratio of the two in the body is significant but it's definitely not something to get hung up about. Omega 6 fats should outnumber omega 3 by a ratio of 4:1 but at present it is more like a ratio of 25:1 due to us eating more vegetable oils like sunflower oil, corn oil, eggs and meat. By simply increasing the amount of omega 3 containing foods in our diet we can help to correct the imbalance.

Omega 3 and the Mediterranean Diet

A Mediterranean diet containing plenty of fruits, vegetables, fish, unsaturated fats such as olive oil, nuts and seeds includes more omega 3 than the western diet eaten by many people nowadays which is made up of mainly refined foods, high fat dairy products, processed meats, fried foods, pre-packaged foods, additives, artificial sweeteners and little fruit and vegetables.

A large-scale study showed that a Mediterranean diet significantly reduced the risk of a person being diagnosed with depression compared to those who did not follow these eating habits. So definitely something to think about.

Magnesium

This is a really important and underrated nutrient when it comes to stress, anxiety and depression.

Magnesium works in tandem with calcium to relax muscles. Calcium contracts the muscles and magnesium relaxes them. Therefore, it can help with relaxing muscle tension and help you to unwind.

Magnesium also plays a key role in energy production. Having an adequate magnesium intake can really help to boost energy.

Magnesium also aids sleep and reduces pain in aching joints and muscles.

Clinical trials have shown that magnesium can stimulate the brain's use of a neurotransmitter called GABA (Gama-aminobutyric acid) whose job is to calm down nervous responses, in particular reducing beta waves in the brain associated with analytical thinking, logic and focus. In anxiety sufferers, the beta waves have gone into overdrive which leads to excessive focus, racing mind and fight or flight response, magnesium can help to calm this down.

The RDA for magnesium is 310mg - 420mg for an adult.

Nutritious sources of magnesium include:

Green leafy vegetables

Avocados,

Nuts

Legumes

Seeds

Wholegrains

Dark chocolate

Bananas

Apricots

Calcium

Calcium is important for regulating mood, it's known as one of natures sedatives and helps to calm and relax you. It is required by the body to produce the sleep hormone Melatonin.

It's important to have the correct ratio of calcium and magnesium, too much of one or the other can lead to stress in the body, hence the need to eat a balanced diet.

Nutritious sources of calcium include:

Dairy products

Almonds

Green leafy vegetables

Broccoli

Tahini

Fortified plant-based milk

Parsley

GABA

GABA is an amino acid that is produced naturally in the brain that works as a neurotransmitter. Its' function is to block certain brain signals and decrease the activity of the nervous system enabling us to feel less anxious and in less pain.

Low levels of GABA are linked to anxiety, mood disorders and chronic pain.

You cannot obtain GABA naturally from foods, however, fruits, vegetables and teas influence how GABA works in the brain, so a nutritious diet is important.

Zinc

Zinc manufactures enzymes which are required for serotonin (happy hormone) synthesis and also for the production of GABA (calms nervous responses).

Zinc helps our bodies deal with stress. When we are stressed, we lose zinc from our bodies through urine and sweat.

Animal studies have shown that zinc reduces symptoms of anxiety and depression. Also, clinical studies have shown that zinc levels appear to be low in people who are depressed or anxious.

Nutritious sources of zinc include:

Beef

Crab

Pork

Oysters

Beans

Cashew nuts

Chickpeas

Pumpkin seeds

Walnuts

Prawns

Green leafy vegetables

Lentils

Tofu

Sesame seeds

One day you're going to wake up and realise that some things just don't bother you the way they used to.

B Vitamins

B vitamins are essential to wellbeing. They are a group of vitamins that are generally found in many of the same food sources. As they are water soluble, they cannot be stored in the body so need to be taken in from the diet daily. They are the key components of energy production and support the function of the nervous system.

By eating whole grains, green vegetables, oily fish and meat you should be able to keep your B vitamin levels in good check. Some people opt to take a vitamin B complex supplement too, but make sure to take advice from your medical professional first.

We require all B vitamins in our diet, (we shouldn't take them singularly as a supplement in isolation useless advised to do so by a medical professional) but, the main two to be aware of when it comes to mental health are vitamin B12 (thiamine) and vitamin B9 (folic acid).

Vitamin B12 has been studied greatly over the years in relation to mental health and there is a strong link between low vitamin B12 levels and anxiety and depression.

Vitamin B12 is required for making use of protein and helps the blood carry oxygen, hence it's essential for energy. It's needed for the synthesis of DNA and for nerves. It also helps to deal with toxins in the body such as tobacco.

Nutritious sources of vitamin B12 include:

Oysters (not that we eat them that often!)

Sardines

Eggs

Prawns

Milk

Turkey

Chicken

Cheese

Salmon

Lamb

Fortified products such as soya milk, cereals and marmite.

You may know people or you yourself may suffer from low vitamin B12 levels which has resulted in you feeling depressed and tired.

Some people have injections from the doctor if their level gets too low which helps them to have more energy and lower depression. If you are feeling depressed, tired, suffering from symptoms such as numbness, tingling, palpitations or light-headedness, then this is something worth getting measured by your doctor.

Vitamin B9 (folic acid)

Vitamin B9 has been shown in several studies to be linked with anxiety and depression. It is essential for brain and nerve function.

Vitamin B9 and vitamin B12 are involved in the breaking down of an amino acid called homocysteine. If levels of homocysteine become too high due to low levels of vitamin B12 and Vitamin B9, then this can become toxic to nerve cells. Higher levels of homocysteine have been linked to mental health problems.

Nutritious sources of vitamin B9 (folic acid) include:

Spinach

Broccoli

Lentils

Chickpeas

Avocados

Eggs

Asparagus

Fortified cereals

B VITAMINS

B vitamins are essential to mental and emotional wellbeing. We require them from our diet daily because they cannot be stored in the body like vitamins A and D can.

B vitamins are destroyed by alcohol, refined sugars, nicotine and caffeine hence why some people can become deficient in them.

Including plenty of green vegetables and oily fish can help. Taking a vitamin B complex supplement can also be helpful but always take professional advice first regarding supplementation.

Iron

Iron is required for the production of red blood cells and for oxygen transportation in the blood.

Iron deficiency is reasonably common, especially if you are vegan or vegetarian.

Iron helps to keep your mood steady and low levels have been shown to result in neurons slowing down, leading to anxiety, depression, poor concentration and restlessness.

Nutritious sources of iron include:

Green leafy vegetables

Beans and lentils

Figs

Dried apricots

Dates

Pumpkins seeds

Liver

Red meat

Spirulina, I don't much like the taste of spirulina but if it's your thing then go for it!!!

Selenium

Selenium plays a crucial role in metabolism and thyroid function. It also protects the body from free radical's and carcinogens which can cause damage to living cells. It helps to boost the immune system and slow down age-related mental decline.

Studies have shown that levels too high or too low can put you at risk of depression.

One of the most reliable sources of selenium is brazil nuts, other nutritious sources include:

Turkey

Tuna

Brown rice

Sunflower seeds.

Vitamin E

Vitamin E is best known for its antioxidant properties and works well with selenium to protect against disease and promote healing. There has been some research that shows that low levels of vitamin E are linked to depression. But, before you go and consume too much there are negative effects from over consumption of vitamin E, so stick to the daily recommended amount of 12 mg.

Vitamin E levels have also been measured to be lower in depressed patients compared to healthy volunteers.

More research needs to be done in this area to work out the association between vitamin E and depression.

Nutritious sources of vitamin E include:

Sunflower seeds

Peanuts

Sesame seeds

Almonds

Tuna

Sardines

Sweet potato

Olive oil

Whole grains

A bird sitting on a tree is never afraid of the branch breaking, because its trust is not on the branch but on its own wings.

Always believe in yourself.

Don't Be Scared It's not as Hard as You may Think!

If you look at the food sources of the various vitamins and minerals listed on the pages in this chapter you will see that many of the same foods keep being repeated. Hopefully, this will give you some confidence and reassurance, knowing that it's not as difficult as you may think to obtain all the nutrients that you require to improve your mental health and general wellbeing.

To boost and maintain our mental health we need to eat a diverse and balanced diet containing a variety of different wholegrains, vegetables, fruits, lean meat, fish, nuts, seeds and legumes.

My favourite foods that I began with when I adjusted my diet were:

Brown rice	Oats
Celery	Ginger
Cucumber	Turmeric
Lettuce	Dark Chocolate
Avocado	Kale
Salmon	Cherry Juice (chapter 12)

Cashew nuts

Watercress

Walnuts

Almond milk

Plain soya yogurt

Don't be scared of change,

Change is part of growth.

Raksha

THE MEDITERRANEAN DIET

*A Mediterranean diet is made up of plenty of fish,
vegetables, fruit, beans, whole grains, nuts, seeds and
olive oil. Whereas a western diet is typically made up
of refined grains like white bread and pasta, red
meat, processed meat, fried foods, pre-packaged
foods, high sugar drinks, potatoes and high fat dairy
products.*

*Research following people who eat a Mediterranean
diet compared to a western diet showed that people
who ate a Mediterranean diet had lower incidences of
depression compared to those who ate a western diet.*

We are responsible for our own recovery. Others can assist us along the way, but only we know what we feel inside.

Although it may be tough to hear, we really do need to take onus of our own health and learn what we need to do to get us through each day.

CHAPTER FIVE

Breakfast Time

*Breakfast – the first meal of the day, breaking the
fasting period of the previous night.*

Although food on its own won't necessarily get you
out of depression or anxiety it can definitely help.

I've used it as a tool for many years to help control
and alleviate my own symptoms and often
recommend it to others as it is very effective.

What's most important is that we keep our blood
sugar level stable to help maintain our mood, focus,
concentration and energy levels.

If we combine protein and complex carbohydrates at
breakfast time, we get a slow and steady release of
energy throughout the morning to keep blood sugar
level stable and our mood more balanced.

It is a good idea to eat protein and carbohydrates
together at breakfast time if you can because most
protein-based foods contain tryptophan which is
converted into serotonin the 'feel good' hormone in
the brain.

A lift in insulin in the blood occurs when we eat carbohydrates and this helps the tryptophan to cross the blood brain barrier and enter the brain to be converted into serotonin, hence the need for protein and carbohydrates to be eaten together.

Many meals in this chapter contain protein combined with carbohydrates, they also contain other nutrients which are beneficial for the nervous system and mental wellbeing such as B vitamins (in whole grains, eggs and mushrooms) magnesium (in greens, nuts and seeds), fibre, probiotics, prebiotics and beneficial fats.

STEP FOUR

Be Sure to Eat Breakfast

Every day, (or as often as you possibly can) attempt to eat a good breakfast. Maybe plan what you are going to have for the next few days. Write it down in the log section at the back of this book, so you don't forget.

People who eat a nutritious breakfast tend to overall have better mental health than those who don't.

Nutritious Breakfast Ideas

- Wholemeal toast or gluten free alternative for those avoiding gluten, with peanut butter (or another nut butter) topped with sliced banana or avocado.

- Plain unsweetened live yogurt or dairy free plain yogurt with oats mixed in and some fruit or nuts on the top. *I always keep blueberries*

*and cherries in the freezer so that I never run
out of fruit and a tub of oats in the cupboard.*

- Porridge made with either milk, nut milk, soya milk or oat milk, topped with chopped nuts and a little maple syrup, fruit or honey and a sprinkle of mixed seeds.

- Scrambled or poached egg on wholemeal bread, sourdough or gluten free bread.

- Mushroom Omelette and watercress.

- Avocado on toast topped with kimchi.

- Fortified low sugar cereals such as Weetabix, Shredded wheat, Bran flakes, All-Bran, add some chopped up fruit or seeds for added nutrients.

- Avocado smoothie - 1 small avocado, 1/3 cucumber sliced, juice 1/2 a lemon, water. All placed in a blender.

DAIRY – SOMETHING TO THINK ABOUT

You may have noticed that I mention dairy and gluten free alternatives within my meal ideas. My reason for this is firstly, that during my own recovery journey I homed in on the fact that my symptoms were often exacerbated by dairy, gluten, refined sugar, caffeine and alcohol, but in particular dairy products. This was also the case for one of my children who has attention deficit disorder.

I'm not telling you to necessarily go down this route, but if you feel that certain foods may be triggering your symptoms or would like to see if certain foods effect your mental health, eliminate the food or food group that you suspect for two weeks and keep a diary of how you feel.

If you notice a change in your mental health discuss with your doctor or nutritional expert about removing it from your diet. It's important to discuss it with a professional especially if it's a whole food group such as gluten or dairy products.

If you decide to remove foods from your diet, make sure that you are still consuming a wide variety of foods and not being overly restrictive and consuming alternative sources of vitamins and minerals that you may be missing out on by removing them.

I tread with caution though when discussing this and personally don't advocate that everyone should go down this route because elimination diets can lead to nutritional deficiencies and disordered

eating if you're not careful.   Those with eating disorders should seek professional advice.

The use of the Mediterranean diet can help in the reduction of depressive symptoms, but because the effects of diet varies from person to person, you would need to see for yourself how dietary changes affect your own mental wellbeing.

I look forward to what may unfold in the future regarding this research area and really hope that this type of approach may become a more recognised management tool along side other methods.

OATS

Oats are a great source of vitamins, minerals, fibre and antioxidants. They contain an antioxidant called avenanthramides which may help lower blood pressure. They also contain a type of soluble fibre called beta-glucan which reduces cholesterol, prevents blood sugar peaks which helps maintain a more level mood, increases the feeling of fullness and they also feed the good bacteria in the gut which are beneficial to mental health.

"Take care of your body. It's the only place you have to live."

Jim Rohn

Every day is a new beginning.

Take a deep breath and start again.

CHAPTER SIX

The Importance of a Healthy Gut

Gut health and Mental Wellbeing

Although there is still a lot more research to be done in this area, there is a growing body of evidence linking diet and gut health to mental health and wellbeing.

Our gut and brain are able to communicate with each other. They communicate through our nervous system, blood system and the immune system.

The vagus nerve which travels from the brain stem to the abdomen is the primary channel of information between the hundreds of millions of cells in the gut and our central nervous system. It controls many of the bodily processes that we are not even aware of, such as maintaining heart rate and controlling digestion.

Within our gut live up to 1000 different bacteria, these along with the other microorganisms such as fungi and viruses that live there make up what is known as our gut microbiome. The gut bacteria help us in many ways, but disruption of their populations through poor diet, stress, medication and environmental toxins can potentially contribute to problems including anxiety and depression.

It's not as simple as saying improve your gut microbiome and all your symptoms will disappear but, doing so can really improve your situation. I will be explaining how you can do this in due course, so stick with me!

If we eat a diet which is low in nutrients, containing a lot of processed foods, refined sugar, alcohol, red meat and low levels of fruit, vegetables, oily fish, nuts, seeds and legumes we can negatively change the populations of the so called 'good bacteria' in the gut.

If this happens, the lining of the gut wall can become damaged as the populations of the good bacteria are not present to enable the tissues to be repaired. This leads to gaps appearing in the gut wall and leaks start to appear.

By the gut walls becoming more porous they can allow pathogens to squeeze through into the blood stream. Immune cells follow them into the blood system and this triggers off inflammation.

Inflammation signals to your brain that something is wrong in the body, we begin displaying sickness behaviour and seek a nice quiet place in the warm to recover, such as in bed. This is frequently in people with depression. It is believed that reducing inflammation in the body could reduce depressive and anxious symptoms.

It's time to trust my instincts, close my eyes and leap!

Wicked

The Western Diet and Our Gut Microbiome

Many of us eat what is called a western diet, a diet that is high in processed and refined foods such as pasta, white bread, processed meats, sugary breakfast cereals, biscuits, cakes, ready meals and other convenience foods but low in fibre, fruits, vegetables, fish, nuts, seeds and legumes.

Studies have linked the western diet with a number of health issues ranging from heart disease, autoimmune disorders, and cancer to anxiety, depression and other mental health conditions.

Apart from the diet being low in fibre and fresh fruit and vegetables another big problem with it is that it is not very diverse, with the same foods tending to be eaten over and over again. To have a healthy gut microbiome we need to eat a varied diet, full of lots of different nutrient dense foods.

One diet that has been shown to reduce symptoms of depression is the Mediterranean diet, which is high in fibre, vegetables, fruit, fish, legumes, nuts, seeds and extra virgin olive oil.

To improve the health of your gut there are a number of things that you can do:

Firstly, move from a western diet to a more Mediterranean diet.

Include more	Avoid too much
Fish	Refined sugars
Vegetables	Fried foods
Fruit	Processed foods
Nuts and Seeds	Alcohol
Olive oil	Artificial sweeteners
Legumes	Red meat

Add the following into your diet:

- **Prebiotics.** These foods help maintain the lining of the gut and keep it strong. The fibre in these foods is difficult for the body to digest. They resist digestion in the small intestine and reach the colon, part of the large intestine, where they are fermented by bacteria producing a substance called butyrate. A function of butyrate is to help to repair the gut lining. Prebiotics are foods such as pulses, onions, garlic, leeks, sweet potatoes, chicory, mushrooms, bananas and celery.

- **Polyphenols.** Compounds found in plants which help to prevent damage to cells within the body. Foods containing polyphenols include, green tea, dark chocolate, red onions, blueberries, sage, rosemary and olive oil.

- **Probiotics**. These are live bacteria which are beneficial for your digestive system. Foods containing probiotics include live yogurt (dairy free options are available just watch out for the sugar content), sauerkraut, kefir, kombucha and some cheeses such as Gouda, Mozzarella and Cheddar.

  Probiotics help us to absorb calcium and magnesium, two minerals which are very important for the management of stress and anxiety. Probiotics synthesise certain vitamins in the intestines, for example, several of the B vitamins including vitamin B12. These vitamins are vital for the functioning of the nervous system and for converting food into usable forms of energy.

- **Vitamin D.** There is connection between low levels of vitamin D and low mood. Having low levels of vitamin D is not good for your microbiome and is connected to inflammation in the body.

  Research has shown that low levels of vitamin D are linked to depression and other mental health problems. To increase your vitamin D levels, get out in the sunshine, eat more mushrooms and eggs and take a supplement in the winter.

The recommended daily dose for a vitamin D supplement is somewhere between 10-25 micrograms for an adult.

- **Omega 3.** The western diet contains high quantities of Omega 6 fatty acids obtained from margarine, sunflower oil, fatty meat and dairy products. These types of fats are inflammatory. This type of diet also contains low levels of omega 3 fatty acids, which are anti- inflammatory.

  Omega 3 fatty acids called EPA and DHA found in oily fish are precursors to a group of compounds called prostaglandins which regulate the anti-inflammatory response in the body.

  By eating more omega 3 containing oily fish such as salmon, mackerel, herring, tuna (not tinned) and sardines we can cause our bodies to produce more anti-inflammatory compounds and potentially reduce the levels of inflammation in the body which is beneficial to brain health amongst other things.

  If you do not eat fish, then taking an Omega 3 supplement made from algae would be beneficial.

- **Resistant Starch.** Foods containing resistant starch are not easily absorbed by the body and reach the large intestine where they feed the bacteria there forming a substance called butyrate as mentioned earlier, which protects the gut membrane. Remember a healthy gut membrane is essential to better mental wellbeing.

Foods containing resistant starch include, bananas, peas, lentils, chickpeas and potatoes which have been cooled down.

Mushrooms contain fibre, B vitamins and vitamin D. Mushrooms contain an amino acid called ergothioneine which helps reduce inflammation. Eaten raw mushrooms contain high levels of prebiotic oligosaccharides which feed friendly bacteria in the gut.

Other things which you can do to improve your gut microbiome include:

- Cut down on your use of antibiotics, only take them if you really need them.

- Open your windows every day to change the air.

- Get out in nature.

- Own a dog (but only if you have the time and money to look after it) or spend time with animals. Evidence has shown that people who own or have contact with dogs have healthier microbiomes.

- Reduce your stress levels, learn to take time out, relax, meditate, do a sport or hobby you enjoy.

- Don't compromise on sleep. Sleep is very important. Refer to chapter thirteen and step thirteen.

- Avoid using antibacterial soaps and cleaners too much as they kill the beneficial bacteria on the surface of the skin.

Our gut bacteria help us in many ways.

Disruption of their populations through poor diet, stress, medication and environmental toxins can potentially trigger or exacerbate anxiety and depression.

CHAPTER SEVEN

Being Mindful

(Incorporating Mindfulness into Your Day)

Mindfulness

What's it all about?

Being mindful is about living completely in the NOW.

It's about noticing this second, how you feel, what you think and what you want without criticism or judgment.

To practice being mindful we focus on what we can **hear, see, touch, smell and taste** in the present moment.

It has been shown that practicing mindfulness regularly can calm the nervous system and reduce symptoms of anxiety and depression.

When you drink just drink,

When you walk just walk.

Zen saying

Mindfulness and Meditation

Everyone you speak to these days seems to be telling you to be mindful or meditate in order to feel better.

It is true that meditation and mindfulness do have an amazingly positive effect on our mental health when practiced regularly.

They help to calm the mind, reduce symptoms of mental illness, reduce pain and increase concentration. The problem is when we feel stressed and anxious, we often feel that we can't sit or focus to engage in them no matter how hard we try.

One way to incorporate being mindful into your day is to practice being mindful whilst doing an everyday activity such as brushing your teeth, having a shower, eating or drinking.

When we practice being mindful whilst doing daily activities, we take time to focus on what things look like, how they feel, any sounds you may be hearing, what something may taste like and how it smells.

The aim of the practice is to notice when our mind gets distracted and is taken away from focusing on these sensations, then if or when we notice this, gently bringing our attention back to focusing on the moment without criticising ourselves.

Take a moment to be mindful right now.

What can you

See

Hear

Touch

Taste

Smell

What Is the Difference Between Mindfulness and Meditation?

Mindfulness and meditation have many similarities, but they are not exactly the same thing.

Meditation tends to be, (although not always) a more formal seated practice where you focus inwards to increase calmness, concentration and emotional balance. It usually begins by bringing your awareness to your breath and then consciously guiding your mind towards an anchor or a single point of focus.

In meditation you tend to spend a specific amount of time during which you are tuned inwards.

Mindfulness is the simple act of paying attention and being present in whatever you are doing. When most people go about their daily lives their minds tend to wander. When we are being mindful, we are actively involved in the activity that we are doing with all our senses. If our mind does wander, we gently bring it back to what we are doing.

Mindfulness can be practiced anytime, it supports meditation. Meditation expands mindfulness.

Mindfulness is the awareness of something, whereas meditation is the awareness of nothing.

"You can't stop the waves, but you can learn to surf."

Jon Kabt-Zinn

"The mind is like water. When it's turbulent, it's difficult to see. When it's calm, everything becomes clear."

Prasad Mahes

Applying Mindfulness to Your Everyday Life

Shower time can be the perfect time to practice being mindful and to calm your mind down before the day begins.

Focusing on the sensations in the shower can give us a break from our stressful and anxious thoughts and lower stress hormone levels in the body.

These effects can last long into the day.

If you give your shower time your full and undivided attention you can bring an element peace to your day.

If time is short you can use the same principles when brushing your teeth or hair, washing your face, having a cup of tea or even sitting on the bus.

Remember, all you need to do is focus on what you can see, hear, touch, taste and smell.

STEP FIVE

Taking a Mindful Shower

Turn on the shower, feel the sensation of the water on your hands and sound of the water running.

Step into the shower.

Feel your feet on the ground.

Do you feel centred and grounded?

Feel the temperature of the water on your skin. Is it hot or cool?

Notice the sound of the water.

Notice your breath.

What can you feel in your body? Do you have any aches and pains, if so just notice them.

How does the water smell?

Can you hear the water hitting the shower base or bath and travelling down the plug hole?

Now pick up the soap or shower gel, how does it feel?

Focus on the smell of the soap. Notice how it feels when you rub it onto your skin.

Watch the water flow over your skin and wash the soap from your body and disappear.

Notice your breath, and the feel of your feet on the floor.

Towards the end of your shower as the water hits your head and flows over your body, visualise a white light covering your body, then as you breathe in, allow the light to fill your body with white light and positive energy.

TIP:

Citrus smells work well for reliving stress and anxiety.

I find it helpful to use shower gels and shampoos which are either lemon, orange or bergamot scented to improve my mood and reduce my anxiety levels.

I also find it beneficial to have a citrus scented hand soap, so I get exposure to a citrus scent during the day.

"I was always looking outside myself for strength and confidence, but it comes from within. It was there all the time."

Anna Freud

STEP SIX

Write down your daily goals

What Are Your Goals for Today?

Write down what you want to achieve today and how long you want to spend on each activity. Be realistic. This can help to clear your mind and help you to feel less weighed down and more focused.

You may need to redo your list several times during the first few days that you do it, as it's common to overestimate what you can achieve.

The aim of the exercise is for you to be honest about what you can cope with, but also to take away some of the pressure and anxiety associated with trying to remember what it is you have to do.

This process can give you a boost as it helps you to be more focused and you get to see what you have achieved, but it can also identify where you may need help and assistance which is a positive thing.

Use the log section to write down your goals and the effect that doing this has had on you.

CHAPTER EIGHT

Our Internal Critical Voice and Acceptance

When our internal critical voice is on overdrive it can be particularly distressing, criticising and commenting on everything we do, telling us we are no good, that we're ugly, unemployable, going to deteriorate or are stupid or boring. Our natural reaction is to ignore it, try and distract ourselves from it or push it to the back of our minds. But this only serves to make it go on at us even more and become more persistent.

Something that I've found particularly helpful is to accept this internal voice, stop fighting it. *This voice is only a small part of us not the whole of us (even though it feels bigger than it actually is).* Respect it, let it speak, you do not need to act on it, just listen to it without judgement, rather than pushing it away.

This may sound strange but, by allowing it to speak you give other parts of your mind the opportunity to contribute to the internal discussion, hopefully enabling you to find a level of balance and calmness, as areas of your mind work together rather than against each other.

When we are battling with critical thoughts the thoughts often get louder and louder until we listen like a toddler pulling on our trouser leg when they want something.

Accepting them isn't an act of giving in, it is quite the opposite, it places you in a more powerful position, a position where you can make choices, have a say and shape your own life.

For example,

If you were having the thought that you were useless, that you weren't going to amount to anything, you would notice the thought, allow it to be there,

maybe thank your mind for that thought,

notice how it makes you feel.

Where in your body you feel any sensations that it brings up, such as butterflies in your stomach or a lump in your throat.

Then pause for a second and breathe into that area.

Following this allow the thoughts and feelings that are present to just flow past, maybe attached to a stick flowing down stream or a leaf falling off a tree.

The temptation when you get these kinds of thoughts would be to act on them, possibly in a negative way against yourself, maybe through self-harm, compulsions, addictive behaviours or avoiding situations, because they are making you anxious or angry. But by just sitting there and allowing the thoughts to be there without acting on them or getting attached to them you take away much of their power.

This isn't an easy process to do at first because you often react without thinking or the anxiety of sitting with the thought can be quite overwhelming. Therefore, you should only sit with what you can cope with.

What often happens if you do take time to sit with these thoughts when they arise and accept them for what they are actually are which is 'just thoughts', is the intensity of the feelings peak, then they naturally decrease and reach a natural balance. The more you practice this when difficult emotions arise the easier it becomes.

This process allows you to be less attached to the past and not as fearful of the future, both of which are common causes of anxiety. It enables you to live in the present and make choices over your life rather than being driven by anxiety and fear. This ultimately can expand the world that you are living in and enable you to take on new things if you want to because you are more able to deal with emotions that come up when you take new steps.

BEING AN INTROVERT IS NOT A BAD THING

You feel like you don't fit in.

You worry that you struggle to mix.

You hate large groups of people.

You can't stand meaningless conversation.

You feel others don't get you.

You'd rather sit in a coffee shop and watch people go by.

You worry but, it is society that says we should be more extrovert, more confident and more outgoing.

This is not true!

There is room for all types in this world, extroverts, introverts, extroverted introverts and introverted extroverts or whatever else you want to be. Trying to be someone you're not, will make you unhappy.

It's ok to be quiet, it's ok to be chatty.

Remember you are ok just as you are.

Be proud!!!

"Accept - then act.

Whatever the present moment contains, accept it as if you had chosen it.

Always work with it not against it.......This will miraculously transform your whole life."

Eckhart Tolle

little by little

day by day

When you're tired, don't quit, just rest.

Remember to take a deep breath.

STEP SEVEN

Prepare Snacks for the Day Ahead

This sounds like a no brainer, but most of us forget to do this. But not anymore!

Making sure you plan ahead and have some snacks available to eat mid-morning to keep your blood sugar balanced really helps to maintain mental clarity and reduce anxiety.

Examples of snacks could include:

Nuts

Chopped up vegetables like carrots, peppers, celery or cucumber with houmous.

Oat cakes.

Apple with peanut butter

Hard boiled eggs

Fruit such as pineapple, watermelon or banana

Having some snacks to hand will prevent you from reaching for sugary foods and caffeinated drinks which will help to keep your mood balanced and reduce anxiety.

CELERY

Celery is a brilliant snack with peanut butter or houmous, it contains a compound called 3-n-butylphthalide which acts as a pain killer. It may not be as long lasting as over the counter pain killers, but it does have a positive effect. It also contains a group of chemicals called coumarins which help stimulate the lymphatic system. They help to increase the uptake of excessive fluids by the lymphatic system and also aid the removal of excess fluid from the body.

TIP:

I've found that just eating a couple of sticks of celery in the morning has made a difference to my pain and anxiety levels in the short term. I always carry some around with me to snack on during the day.

(If you're not keen on celery I've found eating cucumber sticks are also helpful).

It takes a little patience, takes a little time. A little perseverance and a little uphill climb.

Dear Evan Hansen

CHAPTER NINE

It's Lunch Time

The Importance of Eating Regularly

How many times has it got to lunch time and you are too busy to get something to eat or feel too low or tired to be bothered to make anything? I couldn't possibly count the number of times that I have left planning lunch too late only to end up either having nothing to eat or quickly boosting my energy with a quick chocolate bar or ready-made sandwich.

Although it is ok to do this every once in a while, to keep our mood more stable and our brains thinking more clearly and for longer it's helpful to have more nutrient dense lunches.

Something that I often say to people is that it's not the foods that you are eating that are necessarily the problem, it's the important nutrients that you are missing out on when you are eating more convenience and processed foods that cause the problem.

By eating more nutritious foods at mealtimes you tend to have less room for 'junk' foods but also you will be more satisfied by what you've eaten and less likely to crave less nutrient dense foods.

However hard it may seem at first, it is beneficial to our mental wellbeing to make time in the middle of the day for a break and some lunch.

Step 8 shows some nutritious meal choices.

If you are out and about, plan ahead and take some lunch with you.

Part of the aim to feeling better as mentioned in Chapter 5 is to keep your sugar levels as balanced as possible to stabilise your mood and maintain energy levels. Missing lunch is only going to cause your blood sugar levels to dip affecting your mood, causing fatigue, anxiety and loss of concentration.

Slow Release Carbohydrates Over Fast Release Carbohydrates

Try to avoid eating fast release carbohydrates where possible at this time of day, such as white bread, white rice, pasta, biscuits, cakes and pastries as this sends you on a sugar rollercoaster.

When you first eat fast release carbohydrates you can feel great for a short period of time as your blood sugar increases, but after a short amount of time your body responds by secreting insulin, this causes your cells to take up the extra sugar (glucose) from your blood and as a result your blood sugar comes crashing back down again making you feel irritable, tired and foggy headed, sound familiar?!!!

Therefore, it is better to lean towards eating more protein and slow release carbohydrates for lunch. You could achieve this by including foods such as chicken, fish, eggs, chickpeas, lentils, beans, wholemeal bread and pasta, brown rice and vegetables.

May be start by swapping your white bread or pasta for wholemeal and see how you feel.

STEP EIGHT

Lunch Ideas

Some Simple Lunch Ideas Include:

- ### Jacket sweet potato and houmous

  Jacket sweet potato (or potato if you'd rather).
  Cook the night before and reheated to save
  time, top with houmous and some chopped red
  onion with a side salad of lettuce, tomato and
  cucumber.

  *Alternatively, choose whatever greens and
  salad foods you like, such as watercress,
  spinach, red and white cabbage. All will help
  improve gut health and greens, in particular
  will give you a magnesium boost.*

- ### Mackerel and Quinoa

  Precooked mackerel, Precooked sachet of
  quinoa (cooking your own can keep the cost

down) and a green leafy salad, diced red onion, sweetcorn.

- **Tuna salad**

  Tinned tuna, spinach leaves, chopped cucumber, sweetcorn, tomato, olives, red pepper. drizzled in a simple salad dressing of lemon juice and olive oil.

  Serve with some brown rice.

- **Turkey sandwich:**

  Wholegrain bread or rolls.

  Add turkey, avocado, lettuce and sliced tomato.

  Protein such as turkey contains tryptophan which is converted in the brain to serotonin. The wholegrain bread helps it to enter the brain where this conversion takes place.

- **Jacket Potato and Chilli**

  Jacket potato with left over bean chilli from dinner the night before, Chilli recipe is in Step Ten.

- **Peanut butter and sliced banana sandwich** (or on toast).

- **Brown Rice Salad**

  Use either precooked brown rice in a sachet or cook your own and allow to cool. Top with spinach leaves, sliced avocado, chicken, cheese or vegan cheese and tomato salsa.

  Salsa: mix together peeled, deseeded and chopped fresh tomato, diced red onion, finely chopped chilli, clove of garlic some fresh chopped coriander and some salt to taste.

- **Scrambled egg (or scrambled tofu) on wholemeal toast, with watercress.**

Very Quick Lunches!!

- Oat cakes with cashew or peanut butter, cucumber. An orange and some grapes.

- Rice cakes with houmous and chopped carrot sticks. Plus, a pear and some dark chocolate.

- Stir fries are great, there is no shame in buying them either, I do it all the time. Add some toasted cashew nuts, soy sauce or tamari and some brown rice and you have a nutrient dense lunch.

If you are buying your lunch out, consider including some of the following:

- Wholemeal or wholegrain sandwiches rather than white bread containing chicken, turkey or falafels over bacon, salami or other processed meat.

- Vegetable sticks and houmous.

- Fruit pots rather than chocolate bars and sweets.

- Salads without white pasta or heavy dressings.

- Sushi.

- Hard boiled eggs and spinach pot.

- Soups.

- Look in the fruit and vegetable section as sometimes there are small pots of quinoa salad, green leafy salads, chopped vegetables, cooked chicken, nuts and seeds that you can mix together yourself.

- Buy water instead of fizzy, sugary and diet drinks or try herbal teas.

Stay positive

Stay fighting

Stay brave

Stay ambitious

Stay focused

Stay strong

STEP NINE

Afternoon Snack

It's very common to become tired and lethargic mid-afternoon.

A small snack can help keep your mood more buoyant and stop your energy levels wavering. Remember if your energy levels are all over the place it is harder to manage mental health symptoms such as anxiety, depression, intrusive thoughts and mood swings.

Try snacks such as:

Bananas

Sunflower seeds

Strawberries

Celery and peanut butter

Yogurt and chopped fruit

Vegetables and houmous

Watermelon

Nuts

TIP:

If you are feeling anxious, maybe you're waiting to see the dentist, go on the bus or even get out of the front door, try this simple tapping tip.

Tap gently on the side of one hand, the point where you would do a karate chop with the first three fingertips of the other hand.

Now whilst still tapping, take deeps breaths. In through the nose and out through the mouth.

Do this for as long as you need to.

STEP TEN

Dinner/Tea

(evening meal)

I call it tea some people call it dinner! Whatever term you use here are few examples of hassle-free meals you can have for your evening meal to help you on your journey to better mental wellbeing.

In this step I have included some meals that are very easy and require no cooking at all, whilst still giving plenty of nutrients to effectively support your mental health. There are also some simple recipes that can be made in bulk and stored in the fridge or freezer for another day. They are ideal if you are a busy person or your mental health dips at times for whatever reason.

Again you'll probably notice that I've combined proteins and carbohydrates a lot as with previous meals, but also I've used it as an opportunity to sneak in many extra nutrients that are important to our wellbeing such as a variety of vegetables, plant based proteins such as chickpeas, lentils and beans, herbs and spices, foods containing omega 3 such as oily fish and resistant starch, found in potatoes, lentils and chickpeas. A combination of these foods together helps to build a stronger internal system within the body to help you stay mentally well.

Salmon and Quinoa Salad *(serves 2)*

Adding oily fish to your diet several times a week gives you a good source of omega 3. Omega 3 helps to support the nervous system, reduce inflammation and has been shown to reduce depressive symptoms.

Ingredients:

2 salmon fillets (Cooked)

2 tomatoes

½ cucumber

½ red onion

1 clove garlic (crushed)

1 red pepper

1 pouch precooked quinoa

Lemon juice

Olive oil

Chop the tomatoes, cucumber, red onion, garlic and red pepper into small pieces and mix with the pre-cooked quinoa.

Place the mixture on a bed of spinach leaves.

Drizzle over a little olive oil mixed with lemon juice.

Serve with a cooked salmon fillet.

Tuna, Brown Rice and Salad *(serves one)*

Ingredients:

1 tin of tuna

1 bag of mixed salad leaves or watercress

1 tomato

1 cup of broccoli cooked and cooled

2 tbsp cooked brown rice

Fresh chilli

Olive oil

Use either tinned or cooked fresh/frozen tuna. Make a green salad or buy a bag of mixed salad leaves. Watercress works very well with tuna.

Place the green salad and broccoli on a plate.

Add a sliced tomato on the top.

On top of the tomato and salad place a couple of tablespoons of cooked brown rice.

Finally add the tuna on the top.

Chop some fresh chilli and mix with a little olive oil and drizzle over the top.

Chicken, Avocado and Tortilla Salad

(serves one)

Ingredients:

1 chicken breast

¼ iceberg lettuce

¼ cucumber

¼ red onion

¼ avocado

75ml olive oil

1 green chilli

1 clove garlic

1 tbsp honey

Juice of 1 lime

Handful fresh coriander

Chop the chicken breast into small pieces and fry in olive oil.

Add to a bowl of chopped iceberg lettuce, sliced cucumber, finely chopped red onion, 1/4 sliced avocado.

To make the green salsa, place 75ml olive oil, 1 green chilli, 1 clove of garlic, 1 teaspoon honey and the juice of 1 lime in a blender.

Drizzle the green salsa over the top.

To the finished salad add a handful of tortilla chips.

Omelette *(serves one)*

Ingredients:

2 eggs

8 mushrooms

Handful of spinach

Handful of watercress

Olive oil

Vegan cheese (or cheddar cheese)

Place 2 eggs in a cup and whisk them up a little.

Slice the mushrooms and cook in olive oil in a frying pan. When almost cooked add a good handful of spinach.

Once the spinach has cooked down pour over the egg and fry until cooked.

Sprinkle on a little grated cheese or vegan cheese.

Serve with a good handful of watercress.

You can use any vegetables you like, others you could try are courgettes, peppers, onion, broccoli and pre-cooked potato or sweet potato.

Bolognaise *(serves 4)*

Ingredients:

1 pack of Turkey mince or 1 tin of green lentils

2 carrots

2 sticks of celery

2 onions

6-8 mushrooms

4 cloves garlic

1 tin of chopped tomatoes

500g passata

1 level tsp of dried basil

1 level tsp of dried oregano

Salt and pepper

Finely dice the onion, celery, carrot and mushroom and cook until soft in a little olive oil in a saucepan.

Crush the garlic and add to the saucepan.

Now add the turkey mince (or lentils) and cook until the turkey is fully cooked.

Pour over the tinned tomatoes and the passata.

Add the basil, oregano, salt and pepper to the pan and bring to the boil.

Simmer the mixture for 20 mins.

Serve with brown rice pasta or whole wheat pasta.

Bean Chilli *(serves 2)*

Ingredients:

2 diced medium onions

1 tin kidney beans

1 tin black beans

4 cloves garlic

1 stick celery finely sliced

200g passata

1 finely chopped chilli

1 tsp chilli powder (extra to taste)

Soften the onions, celery and garlic in a saucepan for about 5 minutes, add the other ingredients and cook for 10 mins. Serve with rice or a jacket potato.

Spicy Lentils *(serves 4)*

A great quick recipe to eat on its own or served with salad, sweet potato wedges, meat or fish.

Ingredients:

2 tins green lentils

3 cloves of garlic minced

1 tsp cumin

1 tsp ground coriander

½ tsp chilli powder

½ tsp turmeric

¼ tsp salt

1 tsp garam masala

2 tsp balsamic vinegar

1 tsp maple syrup

Place all the ingredients into a saucepan and heat stirring well until cooked through.

Jacket Potato or Sweet Potato

Bake a jacket potato or large sweet potato in the oven then fill with any filling you like.

Possible ideas include:

Left-over turkey bolognaise.

Left-over turkey or bean chili.

Tuna and pesto.

Houmous and sundried tomatoes or houmous and chopped onion.

Baked beans and a little cheese.

Vegetable Curry *(serves 4)*

This is a really nutritious recipe that you can store in the freezer in one serving portion sizes for emergency days.

Ingredients:

1 medium diced red onion

3 large potatoes

2 tbsp medium curry powder

1 tin chickpeas

2 carrots

1 small cauliflower

1 tin chopped tomatoes

300ml vegetable stock

Handful of spinach

Peel and cut potatoes into 2 cm cubes. Also peel and slice the carrots.

Place into a pan of water and bring to boil, cook for 10 minutes.

Cut the cauliflower into small florets and add to water and cook for 5 minutes then place in colander.

Place the diced onion into a separate saucepan and fry until soft with a little olive oil.

Add the curry powder and fry for 30 seconds mixing well.

Add tomatoes to the onion and curry powder, mix and cook for a few minutes then add the vegetable stock.

Place the cooked vegetables and chickpeas into the curry sauce and cook for 10 minutes or until the vegetables are soft.

Add a handful of spinach mix into the curry and allow to wilt down.

Serve with brown rice

If you like a hotter curry add some fresh chilli to your taste.

Cauliflower Curry *(serves 2)*

Ingredients:

1 large red onion

2 cloves of garlic, minced

1 red chilli

2 tbsp madras curry powder

1 large cauliflower

2 carrots

300 ml vegetable stock

200g spinach

Finely slice the red onion and place into a saucepan with the garlic and finely chopped red chilli, plus a little olive oil. Cook until the onions have softened.

Add the curry powder and cook for a minute adding a little of the stock if needed.

Add the cauliflower and carrots to the mixture and mix to coat with the spices and cover with the remaining stock. Bring to a simmer and cook until the vegetables are soft.

Add the spinach and allow to wilt down.

Serve with brown rice.

Spicy Sweet Potato Wedges

These are ideal to add to many different dishes such as salads, curries or own their own with houmous and are easy and quick to make.

Ingredients:

Sweet potatoes

Cumin

Chilli powder

Oregano

Wash and cut sweet potatoes into wedges.

Coat the wedges with a little olive oil and then add to them your choice of spices (examples shown below).

Cook in oven at 180°C for approximately 30 minutes until soft.

Spices:

Mix one tsp of ground cumin with ½ tsp of hot chilli powder and tsp of oregano.

Or

Use something like Waitrose Deep South
Cajun Rub.

Pitta Pizzas

I totally love these pitta pizzas. Great for adding fun to your food and provide a stress-free meal if members of your household want to eat differently, which can be stressful, as they can choose their own topping. We have them on Saturday nights or have them cold in lunch boxes for days out.

Ingredients:

Pittas (we tend to use wholemeal or gluten free ones but obviously the choice is yours).

Tomato puree or green pesto.

Grated cheese. I like vegan cheese but again the choice is yours depending on what type of cheese you like.

Diced or sliced vegetables for the topping such as onions, peppers, mushrooms, courgettes, tomatoes, jalapeno peppers, sweetcorn.

Sliced chicken or tinned tuna.

Chicken, Tomato and Vegetable Pitta Pizza

Pre heat oven to 180 ºC

Place the pitta on a baking tray and spread a layer on tomato puree on to it.

Then add your choice of vegetables, I like to use onion, red pepper, sweetcorn and tomato.

Place your either thinly sliced or diced chicken on the top.

Now sprinkle over some grated cheese to cover.

Cook in the oven for approximately 15 mins or until cooked.

Tuna, Pesto and Sweetcorn Pitta Pizza

Pre heat oven to 180°C

Place the pitta on a baking tray and spread a layer of green pesto on the top. I choose to use a vegan pesto, but there are a variety of pesto's available.

Drain a tin of tuna and place an even spreading of the tuna on top of the pesto.

Sprinkle on some sweetcorn and a few jalapeno peppers if you want it spicy.

Now cover the whole thing with a sprinkling of grated cheese.

Cook in the oven for approximately 15 mins or until cooked.

Chicken or Black Bean Fajitas

(serves 4)

Ingredients:

Wholemeal wraps or I like to use sweet potato gluten free wraps.

650g diced chicken

3 sliced red peppers

3 medium onions

2 chillies finely chopped

3 cloves of garlic finely chopped

Finely sliced iceberg lettuce

Grated cheese

Shop bought tomato salsa or use the salsa recipe in the lunch recipe section.

For the guacamole:

1 avocado

1 finely diced red onion

1 tbsp lemon juice

Cook the onion and peppers in a pan with a little olive oil and some water if necessary.

Cook the chicken in a separate pan in a little olive oil then add it to the peppers and onions. (*I cook the chicken and peppers separately so I can cater for vegetarians*).

Add the chilli and garlic and cook through.

Prepare the guacamole by mashing the avocado and mixing in the red onion and lemon juice. If you want to make it spicy add some chilli.

Heat a wrap in the microwave for a few seconds then place the chicken (swap this step for the black bean mixture below for the black bean fajita) and pepper mixture on the top.

Add some guacamole, iceberg lettuce, tomato salsa and some jalapeno peppers, plus a sprinkling of cheese and roll into a wrap to eat.

For the black bean fajita replace the chicken with black beans and brown rice.

To make the black beans:

Mix 1 tin of washed and drained black beans with 1tsp of ground coriander, 4 cloves of minced garlic, pinch of salt a little olive oil and 1 tsp of flaked chilli.

Place the mixture in a sauce and cook until heated right through and beginning to slightly break down.

Then to the beans mix in 3-4 tbsp of hot cooked brown rice and stir.

Assemble the wrap in the same way as the chicken wrap, by heating the wrap in the microwave for a few seconds, adding to it the bean mixture, lettuce, tomato salsa, jalapeno peppers and cheese. Then wrap it all up!

Easy Salad Dressing

(to use on any salad or slaw)

Ingredients:

2 tbsp olive oil

1 tbsp cider vinegar

¼ clove garlic (minced)

Pinch of salt

1 tsp Dijon mustard

Mix all the ingredients together in a bowl or jar and pour over salad.

Easy Pesto Pasta Sauce

Ingredients:

60g finely chopped fresh basil

2 cloves garlic (minced)

Pinch of salt

3 tbsp olive oil (enough to cover chopped basil).

Toasted pine nuts

Mix all ingredients together in a bowl and then pour over cooked pasta and heat until cooked through.

Add some cheese if you like.

ONIONS

Onions contain the compound inulin which works as a prebiotic. Inulin acts as a food source for the good gut bacteria encouraging its growth.

CHAPTER TEN

Our Relationship with Food

Everyone has some sort of emotional relationship with food. You can't eat without emotions playing a part in some way. We have all had different experiences with food during our lives, some may have been positive, some negative and almost all of us have foods that we find comforting. Therefore, our individual relationship with food will be unique to us and vary from person to person. This is a very important point to remember when adjusting our diets and also for doctors to remember too when treating us.

Our socio-economic background plays a large role in the type of diets and eating habits that we have as well as any significant life events or traumas that may have happened to us. Your parent's relationship with food will have impacted your relationship with food as well as the social circles that you mix in.

Often doctors do not even touch on diet when we make an appointment regarding our mental health. I'm really hoping that with increased awareness of the importance of nutrition that this is something that will improve in the near future.

Unfortunately, it is unlikely that your doctor will have experienced very much nutritional education during their training, but to improve our mental wellbeing we need to be treated as a whole not just a collection of symptoms to which different medications are often given and to be treated as a whole our diet plays a big part.

We need to eat to live, therefore diet plays a very significant role in not only our mental wellbeing but also our physical wellbeing. Every positive change that you make today is shaping a more positive tomorrow. It is unlikely that pills alone will tackle any mental health issue in my view and experience. It's best tackled from several angles to reduce risk of setback and relapse, which is why this book contains more than just nutritional tips alone. Remember we are working on the whole of us rather than just one aspect! This can include medication, therapy, diet and other strategies and tools you choose to put in place.

When it comes to changes to a person's diet and nutrition, steps that act positively or negatively for one person may not work for another in the same way. This can be down to a combination of different factors such as genetics, environmental factors, previous health conditions, support structure, life events and so on. Criticising ourselves, criticising others and others criticising us over the way we eat is just not helpful in any way.

When we do not feel well our food choices can often be driven by our emotions. If you reflect to when you were a child your mum, relative or caring friend may have given you a sweet when you fell over to help you to feel better? This may have really comforted you at the time, maybe it stopped you crying but as an adult, now when things go wrong or you get upset you reach for sugary low nutrient dense foods to soothe and calm yourself and pick up your mood. This isn't necessarily a bad thing, but it depends on how often it is occurring and how much say you feel you have in the matter. The coping mechanisms that we learn as children can remain with us for a lifetime unless we retrain them. This can take time and effort but is far from impossible.

What can be helpful sometimes if you feel the need to eat due to an emotional trigger, which remember is totally normal, is to pause, acknowledge the emotions that you are feeling, may be give the emotion a label such as anxiety, anger, sadness, pain or guilt, then accept how you are feeling and allow these emotions to be present without the need to push them away.

Now that you have created this space for yourself, identify other things that you could do during this time which could calm these emotions and help express and process them rather than using food as your only coping mechanism.

You could try the following:

- Listening to music

- Meditation/mindfulness

- Talking to a friend

- Doing something creative such as sewing, painting, drawing, colouring, woodwork or writing.

- Gardening

- Writing down how you feel

- Dancing

- Yoga

- Take a bath

- Singing

- Smell a scent which you find relaxing or uplifting.

- Simply having a rest

I know that sometimes we just want the nice momentary fuzzy feeling that we get when we eat some chocolate, sweets, cakes, crisps or pizza so we can feel comforted and that's ok and certainly very normal and nothing to be ashamed of. But, for overall health we require other coping mechanisms as well for these emotions to achieve more balance in our lives.

If you feel that you are having problems in this area which are affecting your health, then it may be worth seeking help from you doctor or a psychologist.

Another Emotion Surrounding Eating Can Be Fear

Rather than being driven to eat by emotions such as anxiety or anger there are other times when we can be driven by fear and guilt around food, we may worry that what we eat may make us feel worse or that we are not being 'healthy enough' and this can be as big a problem as over eating or eating 'junk foods' and potentially very dangerous.

Social media sometimes exacerbates this problem as some posts create an element of fear around eating certain foods and the perception that you have to eat a certain way to achieve the ideal figure or outcome. Be careful which people you choose to follow and if they make you feel bad about yourself then unfollow them.

When we are driven by our emotions and in particular fear, we can start to feel very preoccupied by what we eat, leading to us restricting what we are eating and sometimes stopping eating altogether. If you are struggling in this way seek advice from your doctor or a psychologist straight away.

Ideally, given time and by being very gentle with ourselves we can feel relaxed around food the majority of the time and not feel panic or guilt stricken if we eat a doughnut or a bowl of ice cream because sometimes this is exactly what we need. This, however, cannot be forced and happens very gradually as we learn what works for us and gradually gain nutritional knowledge on what we can do to keep our mind and bodies as healthy as possible.

Ultimately, it's about having an overall healthy relationship with food and this includes eating chocolate or a takeaway if we choose to and also being able to listen to the needs of our body and make a choice over what we eat rather than being driven by negative emotions in anyway.

Anxiety can feel like a burden.

That doesn't make you a burden.

CHAPTER ELEVEN

Exercise

Everyone Says Exercise More, but How Can I When I Feel so Low and Anxious?

It's proven that exercise helps to lower anxiety and depression, as well as improve mood, pain, concentration, mobility and stamina.

But, how do we exercise more when we feel too low to get out of bed, too anxious to leave the house or be able to join a club or gym?

Firstly, any movement you do is good for you remember this!

So even if you're lying in bed, stretching your limbs, shrugging your shoulders, or pulling your knees to your chest is helpful, anything at all which increases blood flow, stretches and relaxes your muscles is going to have a positive effect, release feel good hormones and decrease anxiety even if today it's only a little.

If all you can manage to do today is stretch, praise yourself for this and set another goal for tomorrow.

We do however sometimes have to give ourselves an extra big push to get out of bed and start moving. It's important to persevere with becoming more physically active as there are many health benefits associated with it which help us to avoid or relieve certain health conditions associated with a sedentary lifestyle.

If you are someone who is struggling to get outside at the moment and you have stairs stepping on and off the stairs for five minutes a few times a day can help to raise your heart rate and boost mood, you don't get the benefits of the outdoors but you still get the health benefits of moving your body, raising your heart rate and possibly your mood and confidence will improve enough to enable you to take on a little more soon now that your body is moving .

If you are able to get outdoors going for a brisk walk for ten minutes means that you have to walk ten minutes back, this totals to a twenty minute walk which doesn't sound as daunting as saying do twenty minutes of aerobic exercise but is exactly the same thing.

Once you get a bit more active you may feel more able to walk further, increase the frequency or join a class or group. Having a buddy to go with can help as it can be quite daunting to go on your own, although some people, myself included like the space to exercise on their own, so don't feel pressured into exercising with others if you do not want to.

Alternatively, you could use exercise or dance DVDs or exercise equipment at home.

GPs are increasingly putting patients in contact with link workers who help them to find activities in the community that suit them, this is known as social prescribing and is useful if you are struggling with mental health issues or chronic conditions and feel isolated, it can really make a difference to a person's quality of life.

CORTISOL

Cortisol is the bodies stress hormone. It is released during stressful situations.

Researchers have observed that cortisol is elevated in patients who are depressed.

We know that stress causes problems in the brain by effecting memory, learning and regulating emotions.

When stress is left unregulated it can cause many problems in our minds and bodies.

Activities such as meditating, exercising, dancing, floating in water, singing or getting a massage can help to dampen down the stress in our lives.

STEP ELEVEN

Increasing your Activity Levels

Pick one activity that you would like to include in your day, it doesn't matter how small or large it is.

Write it down.

Work out how you will best achieve this. For example, does it need to be broken down into smaller chunks to make it manageable?

Work on your chosen activity at YOUR planned pace, not someone else's!

Write down in the log section at the back of the book how you felt during and after this process.

Following this set yourself another goal, it can be continuing with the activity you were doing or a new one and tick it off when you have achieved it.

Keep going and watch your activity levels rise.

If Things go Wrong

If you have a day where things don't work out as planned, don't beat yourself up. Remember you are looking after yourself not punishing yourself. It's totally normal to get knocked off track sometimes and it's how you react during these times that are most important for your recovery.

So, cry if you need to, get annoyed, punch a pillow then continue working on your goal later that day or the next day. Doing a little is better than doing nothing at all. Try and keep the momentum going if you can.

THE DAY I JOINED A CHOIR

Sitting here, thinking back to the time when I decided to step out of my comfort zone completely 4 years ago.

I'm quite a reserved character, but I really wanted to meet more people and increase my activity levels, so I joined a local choir.

It was so scary walking into a room of new people, plus having to sing as well. I didn't know how my body would react to the increase in activity, but it turned out to be one of the best decisions that I've ever made.

It was more than just singing. I gradually made new friends and became part of a community. I moved my body more but in a gentle way, I had to use my brain to learn the words and remember instructions, this helped to ease my anxiety as did just listening to the songs at home whilst I was practising..

It gave me something positive to do at home as I had to learn the songs and any actions for the following week. Just the process of singing and dancing helped me to process emotions in my body and relieve mental and physical tension that I was carrying around.

As a socially anxious person it was a place that I felt at ease because I didn't have to spend time having long conversations with people if I didn't want to because time was taken up singing.

Something that became apparent to me over time was that other people there also had their own quite significant struggles too which was obviously sad but also comforting to know that I was not alone. We supported each other, but not by being negative and depressing but in a positive and healing way.

BE CREATIVE, IT'S GOOD FOR YOU!

Research has shown that being creative is beneficial for our mental and physical wellbeing. Anything from drawing, painting and pottery to writing, dancing and music can help us to have an increased sense of psychological wellbeing.

CHAPTER TWELVE

Offloading - Journaling

It's difficult to know exactly where to put this next step in the book as it will differ from person to person as to when they choose to do it.

When you struggle mentally your head is often so full of problems, scenarios, what ifs, anxieties, negative thoughts about yourself and all sorts of other things that make it impossible to see the 'Wood for the Trees' when you are just simply trying to get on with your everyday life.

What we all need is a way of off-loading some of these worries and thoughts in a way that is not reliant on others being available to help us or listen to us. Talking over what's troubling us is extremely important but, if we are always reliant on other people to help us, we can feel very vulnerable when they are not there especially if we don't have other coping strategies.

One effective way I have found to achieve this is to write a journal.

Writing a journal often sounds boring and too much effort, but it frees up so much time and headspace, relieves anxiety and gives you more energy and a sense of clarity.

If we create some space to write down what's going on in our minds we can begin to think more clearly and make decisions that are out of choice rather than panic or driven by anxiety.

Writing down what's going on in your mind no matter how dark it may be can really help to lift the pressure and enable you to get a better perspective on what's going on in your life.

It doesn't matter how you choose to do this or what time of day. Ideally, it's better to do it frequently to prevent things from building up, but this is for you to decide. Also, don't forget to write down the positive things that are occurring in your life too!

I usually approach writing a journal by finding a time in the day when I can grab about 30 minutes of peace, but you can sit for 5 minutes, the duration is up to you. I then have an A4 pad and just write down how I'm feeling, any of the worries I have no matter how bad they may seem. If there's an area that seems too heavy to go into at that time, I'll leave it for another time when I feel I can handle it or speak to my doctor about it if it's too overwhelming.

Sometimes I find I don't have the mindset to write or the energy, during those times I'll draw or stick in pictures that express what's going on. It doesn't matter how you approach your journal; you just want to get what's going on in your mind onto paper.

STEP TWELVE

Writing a Journal

Find a time in the day that best suits you, it can be at different times of the day if needs be.

Write down how you are feeling today, any thoughts that are going around and around in your head, any concerns, worries or just what you have been up to.

Use words, pictures, paint, or anything else you like that helps you to express yourself on the page.

Make a note in the log section of the affects you feel after writing a journal.

CHAPTER THIRTEEN

Bedtime

Bedtime Routine

The steps in this book that we have worked through so far are automatically setting you up to have a better night's sleep without you even having to think about it. Whether we like it or not what we do and don't do during the day and evening can have an impact on our sleep patterns.

If you are still sleeping badly at the moment persevere as it takes time to undo old habits and for your internal biochemistry to readjust to the changes that we have made so far.

It's no secret that when you suffer from mental ill health that your sleep can be negatively affected, which can go on to further exacerbate the problem, so sleep is an area worth working on.

The good news is that you do not have to make lots of changes in order to start having a positive impact on your sleep.

When I gradually made the changes in this book to my own lifestyle, I found that over time my sleep pattern returned without me having to place any specific focus on it.

The meals and snacks in this book are aimed at increasing levels of protein in your diet (to provide you when they are broken down with amino acids) which are required for sleep, especially an amino acid called tryptophan. Tryptophan is the amino acid required to make the 'happy hormone' serotonin. Without enough serotonin we cannot produce enough melatonin which is our sleep hormone. Increasing melatonin levels will help you to sleep better.

Foods high in tryptophan include:

Salmon

Beef

Eggs

Tofu

Cheese

Milk

Nuts

Turkey

Chia seeds

Pumpkins seeds

However, there is a catch, high tryptophan foods will not boost serotonin levels on their own. High tryptophan foods need to be mixed with carbohydrates to enable the tryptophan to be absorbed into the brain and converted to serotonin. So, the best way to get a serotonin boost is to eat these foods regularly alongside foods such as brown rice, wholemeal pasta and whole grain bread.

SEROTONIN

Serotonin is also known as 5 HT (5 hydroxy tryptamine) or the happy hormone.

It is found in the brain, bowel and blood platelets.

Serotonin is known for promoting good sleep, regulating appetite, promoting memory and helping to promote positive feelings.

Low serotonin levels may leave you feeling anxious, depressed, irritable or aggressive, you may also have sleep issues, decreased appetite, digestive issues and crave sweet and carbohydrate rich foods.

Diet is not the only way to boost your serotonin levels, other ways include:

- Exercise

- Getting out in the sunshine

- Going for a massage

- Improving your gut microbiome

- Think about something that makes you feel good, such as visualising a happy memory or looking at photos of things that make you happy.

STEP THIRTEEN

Getting Better Quality Sleep

As best you can, work on following a good bedtime routine each evening.

Over the next few days, weeks or months work on gradually making changes to your lifestyle like the ones listed below along with the changes you have already made.

Changes to make for improved sleep include:

- Don't eat heavy meals too late in the evening.

- If you fancy a snack have some walnuts, a banana, turkey and lettuce sandwich, glass of milk or a small glass of unsweetened cherry juice as these may help aid sleep.

- Reduce consumption of caffeinated drinks and chocolate especially in the afternoon and evening.

- Avoid using alcohol to help you get off to sleep or as a way of managing stress and anxiety.

- Do something relaxing before bed such as reading, listening to music or watching a program you enjoy (not a horror film!).

- Turn your phone off at least an hour before bed.

- When using your phone or computer in the evening try using blue light filtering glasses. These can help prevent the interference of melatonin production.

- If you suffer with conditions such as anxiety PTSD or attention deficit disorder, consider trying a weighted blanket. Unfortunately, weighted blankets are expensive. What I did to reduce the cost was purchase a blanket that was exceptionally heavy, about 2.25 kg (for a single bed) and although it wasn't one of the advertised weighted blankets it made a really big difference.

- Rather than introduce new steps at this point I've found it easier to repeat some of the morning steps:

  Therefore, have a mindful wash and brush your teeth.

  Relax into bed and do the heart breathing exercise that we covered in step 1 or another breathing exercise of your choice.

- If you do wake in the night, try doing the heart breathing exercise to help you to drift back off.

ALCOHOL

Alcohol can affect our mood. It can trigger anxiety, stress and depression rather than reducing it.

It's not uncommon, particularly after a stressful day for people to sit down with a glass of wine or something stronger to relax, and in the short term the desired feeling of relaxation does occur.

However, drinking heavily regularly can contribute to feelings of depression and anxiety and make stress more difficult to deal with.

Regular drinking lowers levels of serotonin, the good old 'happy hormone', in the brain. This makes it more difficult for us to regulate our mood and for us to have good quality sleep.

Alcohol is another one of those areas where it depends on the individual as to how much alcohol they can consume before it becomes problematic. Some people can drink a little and others none. I'm the latter, I cannot touch a drop! I had to give up drinking alcohol 15 years ago because I had little tolerance to the effects that it caused, but some of my friends can have a little and as long as they don't go crazy, they're fine.

If you are very anxious or depressed, then avoiding it is ultimately the best option, at least until you are feeling more stable.

Self-harm and suicide are a greater risk for people who have drunk alcohol as they lose their inhibitions and sometimes do things that they wouldn't normally do.

If you are feeling very stressed, anxious or depressed think of other things that you could do instead of turning to alcohol as a form of release and relaxation, such as exercise, talking to a friend, breathing exercises, drinking something else non-alcoholic that you like the taste of, having a bath or listening to music.

MELATONIN

Melatonin is a hormone made by the pineal gland in your brain. It regulates sleep wake cycles.

During the day the pineal gland is inactive, but when it is dark the pineal gland begins to produce melatonin. As the levels of melatonin rise in your blood you begin to feel sleepy.

Bright light inhibits the release of melatonin even if the pineal gland is switched on which is why it is important to avoid screen time before bed.

LETTUCE

Lettuce is a source of folate and soluble fibre. It is thought to calm nerves due to the leaves (especially the dark bitter leaves) containing lactucarium which relaxes nerves, reduces palpitations and induces sleep.

Still Finding It Difficult to Sleep?

If you are still having sleep problems, take a glance again at how many caffeinated drinks you are having in a day such as tea, coffee, cola and energy drinks and swap them completely for another type of drink such as:

- Water.

- Rooibos tea which is quite like 'normal' tea.

- Decaffeinated versions of tea and coffee.

- Chamomile or valerian tea especially near bedtime.

- Milk.

- Nut milks.

- Small glass of fruit juice, cherry juice is very good.

- Iced tea, berry teas are also nice when refrigerated.

- Fizzy water with lime or lemon.

- Mint tea if you find your digestive system is affected by your mental health.

- Decaffeinated lattes with oat milk, nut milk or soya milk if you're a coffee shop lover like me!!!!

Also keep check on your alcohol consumption and other things such as how much dark chocolate you may be eating.

If you are taking positive action and still having sleep problems consult your doctor.

Also, Practice Being Kind to Yourself

Change takes time. It's ok to be annoyed and angry that you can't sleep, that's only natural but try and guide the actions that you take to improve sleep in the direction of selfcare, forgiveness and kindness. By doing actions like the ones mentioned in this section and reminding yourself that it's ok to look after yourself I feel confident that you will eventually see an improvement.

Negative Thoughts

If you find that you are constantly barraged with negative thoughts that you are failing, letting yourself down, it's all your fault, that sort of thing, try not to force the thoughts to the back of your mind as they can often come back even more forceful. Allow the thoughts to be there, accept them for what they are. You don't need to enter into an ongoing conversation with them, just let them flow through your mind like a stick flowing down a stream. Momentarily your anxiety may rise as you do this, but it is likely that it will return back to a manageable level given a few minutes.

Also, keep a pad by the bed to write down any worries or ruminating thoughts that come up.

Write down in the log section things that have helped and maybe things that haven't and any changes that you have noticed.

CHERRIES

Sour cherries contain a significant amount of melatonin. A glass of sour cherry juice before bed has been shown to promote better sleep.

Sour cherries also contain antioxidants which help reduce inflammation and pain.

STEP FOURTEEN

Remembering to Check in With Yourself!

This step is very quick but also very important.

When we make changes such as the ones described in this book, we can if we are not careful, become quite strict and regimented with our routine, worrying that if we miss a step or don't do it exactly right or in the right order then we will not improve. This sadly is very common when people have a mental health problem, as they try to control areas in their lives that feel out of control. This can cause problems and lead to people giving up on trying to recover.

Therefore, what we need to do is to sit quietly for a few minutes as often as we choose, tune in with the feelings in our bodies and our minds to just check that we are not being too hard on ourselves, that we are not being too strict or punishing ourselves through negative talk or actions for not being 'perfect' and recovering as quickly as we think we should.

If you recognise that you are being too harsh on yourself or being driven to do the steps because you are too anxious not to, pause and allow yourself to stop, take a step back and see if you have given yourself enough time to adjust to the changes that you have made already before trying to move forward again.

We all want to progress through the steps at the speed of light, but this is not reality. Everyone's recovery journey will be individual to them, some will move quickly, others more slowly, but most will be somewhere in between. Life events will sometimes get in the way and that's just how life is. The main thing is to stick to what you are doing, little and often, be flexible, don't try to be perfect and remember doing something is often better than doing nothing, no matter how small, unless you are wanting to sit and do nothing that is!

We need to leave the 'all or nothing' approach at the front door and praise the perceivably small things because, they are the things that matter the most as they add up to be the big things later on.

Step fourteen may not apply to you at this time and if it doesn't, feel free to skip it, but always keep it in the back of your mind.

Write any thoughts that may arise when you do this in the log section so you can reflect and make the right choices for you.

CHAPTER FOURTEEN
Working with Professionals

When you have a mental health condition it can be very frustrating and sometimes scary. Due, to the fact that you may be struggling you might have to turn to professionals for treatment and support.

One of the problems that we have in this country is that the funding for these services has been dramatically reduced over recent years which means that many people cannot access the support that they require.

If the system is insufficient, how can we get the best we can out of it?

Your Doctor

Before seeing your doctor, write down any symptoms and any thoughts and concerns that you may have, so that if you get overwhelmed in the appointment you have something to refer to.

Don't expect the Doctors to know what you are thinking and feeling, try your best to get your thoughts and feeling across. If there is anything specific you would like them to do ask them because, often if you don't ask you will not get. If they offer you solely medication, ask for what other support may be available such as referrals to people who can get you support in the community and books you could read.

If your doctor is not interested in your lifestyle, and doesn't ask about your diet, social interaction or your sleep, you may wish to seek the opinion of another doctor. Your doctor should treat you as a whole person which means bringing in the physical, mental and social all together.

I cannot reiterate enough though, if you want something do not expect them to read your mind, ask for it. They do not have the time to ask lots of questions. The worse thing they can say is no.

You may find it helpful to get a friend, partner or somebody you trust to come with you and support you at the appointment.

Doctors Receptionist

If you ring up and it's an emergency and there are no appointments available tell them that you have a mental health problem and need to be seen. If you do not feel well enough to contact your doctor's surgery, ask somebody to help you to make the appointment if you have somebody available to do so.

If you are unable to get an appointment, ask the receptionist if a doctor could phone you instead.

Making appointments online is helpful if it's not an emergency as you don't have to use the phone. If you are able to make online appointments in advance to keep on top of things, then try and do so.

Mental Health Services

If you get referred to mental health services there are several different sections depending upon the severity of your condition, your location, how much support you need and your age.

Initially they may refer you to services where you can speak to somebody on the phone or complete an online course.

You may require more one to one or group support, in which case you would be referred for this and the treatment usually takes place over around a 3 months period.

In some areas are there are support groups and short courses you can attend such as anxiety management courses, mindfulness courses, cookery courses for mental wellbeing and support groups for certain conditions.

If your condition is more complex or severe you may go into secondary care services where you will receive treatment such as psychological therapy and support for longer.

Hospitalisation is a last resort. If this does occur remember you still have a voice even if under section.

Waiting lists for treatments such as psychological therapies can vary depending on where you live but can be quite long.

Waiting Lists

If you are put on a waiting list, accept that you may be waiting for a while. If you get worse, which often happens whilst waiting, go back to your doctor.

If you have the contact details for the service that you have been referred to contact them as well. Do not feel embarrassed or worried to contact them, even if the response you get is cold and not helpful, you need to sometimes push for what you need.

Whilst on the waiting list do what you can to support your mental health.

Eat as well as you can and drink plenty of water, even if you have lost your appetite.

Try to get up and dressed every day if you can even if you go back to bed.

Move your body, do simple stretches, step on and off the stairs or go outside for a walk if you can. If you can cope with more exercise than this then do it and try and keep it up but don't overdo it.

Talk about your problems to a trusted friend or phone organisations such as the Samaritans.

If you don't have anybody to turn to write down what you are feeling to get it out of your head.

Try and believe in the possibility that things will get better.

If you have been on a waiting list for more than a few weeks, phone up and find out how long you will need to wait, this may speed up your appointment.

Seeking Your Own Support

There are many sources of support that are available to you whilst you are waiting.

Check with your employer if you are working, they may offer an Employee Assistance Programme which can provide telephone-based counselling and support, many also offer free face to face counselling.

Look for local charities which offer mental health support, such as The Samaritans, Mind, Rethink, and Teens in Crisis. There may also be additional charities and support groups in your local area although this is not that common but worth looking into to.

If you can afford to do so you may also wish to fund your own treatment or if you have Private Medical Cover this may provide you with the support that you require.

Areas which are proven to be beneficial to mental health recovery:

Counselling or Psychotherapy – you can find qualified professionals at **www.bacp.co.uk**

Equine assisted Psychotherapy

Mediation and Mindfulness classes and courses – *if you are on a low income you may be able to find these courses at a discount or free.*

Emotional Freedom Technique (Tapping)

Social Prescribing – professionals put you in touch with support in the community.

Books on Prescription.

Summary of a whole day

From the moment we wake up we are faced with multiple ways from which we can approach life. When we experience mental health problems, we can often feel the number of options and choices we have has become reduced and we become trapped in negative cycles and driven by our emotions.

The fourteen steps in this book highlight natural areas of potential opportunity where you can step in and make changes to your lifestyle without too much disruption which can positively impact your wellbeing.

This book shows you that it is possible for you to regain your power and make choices which can improve your health and ease symptoms by adjusting everyday activities ranging from how you begin your day to what you eat, how you respond to critical self-talk, and how you approach doing activities that suit you, ones which nurture your soul and help you to heal.

The obvious points where we can make a difference are outlined on the next page in each of my steps one to fourteen, but it's worth remembering that during every second of the day you are presented with yet another opportunity to treat yourself either with kindness or as an afterthought.

STEP ONE: Practicing breathing into the heart area as a way of recentring yourself and calming your nervous system before the day begins.

STEP TWO: Taking notice of things in your life that you are grateful for and writing them down. This helps you to focus on what's important in your life and appreciate it.

STEP THREE: Drinking enough water to prevent tiredness, brain fog, lack of energy and changes in mood.

STEP FOUR: Making breakfast choices that help to balance blood sugar levels and mood, such as yogurt with oats and fruit or scrambled egg on wholemeal toast. Including foods which boost our fibre intake and also our intake of B vitamins, calcium, heathy fats, protein, probiotics and vitamin C.

STEP FIVE: Using the principles of mindfulness in the shower as a tool to focus your mind and reduce anxiety. Focus on what you can see, feel, smell, touch and taste. Use scents which trigger you to feel more grounded, calmer, more focused or uplifted depending on how you are feeling. Citrus scents are useful for relieving anxiety and lavender is very calming.

STEP SIX: Planning realistic goals for the day. It's important to be honest about what you feel you can do even if it makes you a little upset because you can't do something yet that you want to. Let's be honest you can't successfully work upwards from an unrealistic starting point! Always praise victories no matter how small!

STEP SEVEN: Preparing simple snacks such as vegetable sticks and houmous or oatcakes and nut butter to maintain balanced blood sugar levels helps to reduce mood dips and anxiety. This step sounds simple and it is, but it is often overlooked when you are busy. The more balanced you can keep your blood sugar levels the better you will feel.

STEP EIGHT: Lunch ideas that our brain will thank us for. In this step there are lunch ideas to cook or make at home and others that are suitable to take out and about, plus a few tips on buying your lunch when you're out. Again, we pay attention to making sure we include important nutrients that we need for our brain to function well, such as Omega 3, fibre, magnesium, B vitamins, polyphenols, prebiotics, protein and resistant starch.

Planning your lunches will help you to get into a rhythm and also help you to identify which types of foods in particular suit the way that YOUR body and mind works and support you to feel better. Remember that one diet doesn't suit all, so you need to be flexible.

STEP NINE: Afternoon snacks that we can have instead of quick sugar fixes. This step is the same as with step seven. Keeping blood sugars level is key, so don't miss checking in with yourself at this point to see if you require a little nutritional boost to get you through the afternoon.

Don't forget to include checking your fluid intake too!

STEP TEN: Evening meal choices that are quick to make. As with step eight, in this step making a plan may help as well as making sure that you always have a few essentials in the cupboard and freezer so that you can prepare something quickly.

There are some very basic meals in this chapter and some which require a little more preparation, but nothing is complicated. Don't be put off by the fact that there may be a few more herbs and spices than you are used to. Once you have them in your cupboard, you'll see that they are easy to use and last for ages.

This section as with the other meals is focused on making sure you get nutrients which will help you to feel healthier mentally and physically.

STEP ELEVEN: Moving your body more and mixing more. Moving is essential to wellbeing as is social interaction. I really urge you to persevere with this step. Paying particular attention to focusing on things that you enjoy, that intrigue you and draw you in, making you want to do and learn more. If you don't have any motivation, still do this step, the motivation doesn't always come first, often it will join you later.

STEP TWELVE: Freeing your mind from clutter with journaling. Writing down what is going around in your mind can literally feel like lifting a big weight from your body and mind, giving you space to focus on what is important to you and make the right choices.

STEP THIRTEEN: Getting better quality sleep. By making a few adjustments to when and what you eat, including activities that relax and interest you and adjusting what activities you undertake such as limiting phone use before bed can make a difference to your quality of sleep.

Keep a note of things that help and those that hinder your sleep to keep you focused, because sleep is very important and one of the first things to go during periods of stress.

STEP FOURTEEN: Remembering to regularly check in with yourself so you can avoid sabotaging your own progress and notice any signs that need to be taken notice of.

Don't overlook this step, it's probably one of the most important steps to help prevent you from going backwards or if you do get a setback it can reduce its severity.

Remember for each step to jot down your thoughts and progress in the log section.

Where to Begin

Begin by picking one step and sticking to it. You may not see much of a change at first, so give it at least three weeks to become part of your routine.

When Will I See Change?

You will most likely need to combine the effects of several steps before things really begin to improve. So be kind to yourself and allow yourself the time and space to really master each step before taking on the next one.

It doesn't matter if it takes one month, one year or longer to work through and master the steps. Stay focused on where you are heading and hold on to the hope that things can and will change for the better.

Good luck with your recovery journey.

Best wishes

Kate

"The moving finger writes; and, having writ, moves on:

Nor all they piety nor wit. Shall lure it back to cancel half a line,

Nor all thy tears wash out a word of it."

the Rubaiyat of Omar Khayyam

Granny Barb's favourite

Seasonal Fruits and Vegetables

Increasing the number and variety of fruits and vegetables that you eat in your diet will have a positive impact on your mental wellbeing.

If you struggle to know what's in season, below is a list of seasonal fruit and vegetables. However, you can obviously buy whatever is available to you in your supermarket and local shops.

January
Apples, Banana, beetroot, Brussels Sprouts, Cabbage, Cauliflower, Celery, Clementine's, Kale, Onions, Oranges, Parsnips, Pears, Swede, Sweet Potatoes.

February
Apples, Banana, Brussels Sprouts, Cabbage, Cauliflower, Celery, Clementine's, Kale, Onions, Oranges, Parsnips, Swede, Sweet Potatoes.

March
Banana, Brussels Sprouts, Cabbage, Cauliflower, Onions, Oranges, Parsnips, Peppers, Sweet Potatoes.

April
Banana, Cabbage, Cauliflower, Onions, Peppers, Potatoes, Spinach, Watercress.

May
Apricots, Banana, Cabbage, Lettuce, Nectarines, Onions, Peas, Peppers, Potatoes, Spinach, Watercress.

June
Apricots, Asparagus, Banana, Blackberries, Cabbage, Carrots, Courgettes, Lettuce, Nectarines, Onions, Peas, Peppers, Potatoes, Runner Beans, Spinach, Strawberries, Tomatoes, Watercress.

July
Apricots, Asparagus, Banana, Beetroot, Blackberries, Cabbage, Carrots, Courgettes, Spinach, Strawberries, Tomatoes, Watercress.

August
Apricots, Banana, Beetroot, Broccoli, Cabbage, Carrots, Celery, Courgettes, Lettuce, Nectarines, Onions, Peas, Peppers, Raspberries, Runner beans, Spinach, Strawberries, Tomatoes, Watercress,

September
Apples, Apricots, Banana, Beetroot, Cabbage, Carrots, Celery, Courgettes, Lettuce, Nectarines,

Onions, Parsnips, Pears, Peas, Peppers, Plums, Raspberries, Runner beans, Spinach, Sweetcorn, Strawberries, Tomatoes, Watercress.

October
Apples, Banana, Beetroot, Brussels Sprouts, Cabbage, Celery, Kale, Lettuce, Onions, Parsnips, Pears, Peas, Peppers, Plums, Runner Beans, Sweet Potatoes, Tomatoes.

November
Apples, Banana, Beetroot, Brussels Sprouts, Cabbage, Celery, Clementine's, Kale, Lettuce, Onions, Parsnips, Pears, Peas, Runner Beans, Swede, Sweet Potatoes.

December
Apples, Banana, Beetroot, Brussels Sprouts, Cabbage, Celery, Clementine's, Kale, Lettuce, Onions, Parsnips, Pears, Swede, Sweet Potatoes.

Log Section

STEP ONE
Breathing into the Heart Area

Write below your experience of taking time to breathe into the heart area or any other breathing exercise that you chose to do.

Some questions you could ask yourself may include:

How did you feel before the breathing exercise?

What did you notice during the exercise?

Was it beneficial?

Was there anything you would change?

Log Page

STEP TWO
Practicing Gratitude

Note down below your experience of writing things down that you feel grateful for.

Did you notice any change in your thoughts?

Did it influence how you felt about the day ahead?

What was positive about the process?

Was there anything negative or that you found challenging?

Log Page

STEP THREE
Stayed Hydrated – Drinking Enough Water

Note down below how incorporating drinking more water throughout the day has affected your mental and physical wellbeing.

Have you noticed any difference in your concentration, mood, tiredness or pain levels?

Have you found any useful ways which prompt you to remember to drink?

Log Page

STEP FOUR
Breakfast Ideas

Write down below the impact including some of the new breakfast ideas has had on your wellbeing.

If you ate breakfasts prior to trying this step what types of foods did you choose?

If you have made changes what type of changes have you made?

How have these changes affected your concentration, anxiety and depression, fatigue levels and overall wellbeing?

Create a list of breakfasts you could choose from. Also identify one that you could easy turn to on very bad days.

Log Page

STEP FIVE
Taking a Mindful Shower

Write down your experience of taking the time out for a mindful shower. Remember you can also use the same process for other activities if you choose such as eating, washing up and walking.

Things you could think about:

How did it feel to think about taking some time out for yourself in this way?

What sort of thoughts and feelings were present in your body and mind before the shower?

What did you notice happening to your thoughts and feeling during the shower?

How did you feel at the end?

Log Page

STEP SIX
Writing Down your Daily Goals

How did it feel to write down your goals, did it help you to focus and achieve what you wanted to?

Did any difficulties arise during this process such as trying to do too much?

If you did have difficulties how did you or how could you overcome them?

STEP SEVEN
Preparing Snacks for the Morning Ahead

How does it feel to eat more regularly?

Have you noticed any change in your mood, anxiety, depression and alertness?

Which snacks have you found that you like and are there any you can turn to in an emergency?

STEP EIGHT
Lunch Ideas

Make a note of your experience of making lunches that are geared to boost your mood.

How easy did you find it?

If there were difficulties how could you make things easier for yourself?

Were there any meal choices that you particularly liked?

Were there any meals that you feel you could turn to in an emergency? If not, can you think of something that would work for you?

Log Page

STEP NINE
Afternoon Snack

How has having an afternoon snack when required affected your mood, anxiety levels and lethargy?

Have you noticed any changes in your concentration?

What were your favourite snacks?

Is there any you feel you could turn to in an emergency?

Log Page

STEP TEN
Dinner/Tea

As this is often one of our main meals and requires a little more effort, it is worth making some notes to refer to in order to keep yourself motivated.

Have you noticed any benefits to eating the types of meals in this chapter?

How have you coped with the meal preparation and cooking?

Did you experience any hurdles? If so, how did you or how could you overcome them or is there anyone else who could support you?

How have your mood, sleep and energy levels been since implementing the changes?

Log Page

STEP ELEVEN
Increasing your Activity Levels

Which activity did you choose to include or increase?

How did you feel that you got on?

How did you feel before the activity and how did you feel after?

Do you have any future goals?

Log Page

STEP TWELVE
Writing a Journal

How does it feel to get what's going around in your mind down on to the paper?

Have you identified any particular methods which help you to express your thoughts such as drawing, painting, writing, brain storming or sticking in pictures?

Log Page

STEP THIRTEEN
Getting Better Quality Sleep

This is a really important step and worth taking the time to really identify what works for you.

How was your sleep pattern before beginning these changes?

Has your sleep changed?

Have you identified anything which hinders your sleep?

Have you identified anything which helps?

Log Page

STEP FOURTEEN
Remembering to Check in With Yourself

Have you managed to regularly check in with yourself and identify any warning signs that you feel that you may need to listen to?

Write your thoughts below.

Log Page

FURTHER READING

Ardel, K. and Wilds, E. (2011). Teaching Mindfulness to Children and Teens.

Bullmore, E. (2018). The Inflamed Mind.

Johnson, S. (1999). Who Moved my Cheese.

Kennedy, P. (2016). Energy EFT for Teenagers.

Williams, M. and Penman, D. (2011). Mindfulness, a practical guide to finding peace in a frantic world.

Liu, C., et al. (2007). Perceived stress, depression and food consumption frequency in the college students of China Seven Cities. Physiology and Behaviour, 92(4).

Yunsheng, M., et al. (2006). Association between dietary fibre and serum C-reactive protein. The American Journal of Clinical Nutrition, 83(4).

Evers, E. A., et al. (2010). The effects of acute tryptophan depletion on brain activation during cognitive and emotional processing in healthy volunteers. Current Pharmaceutical Design, 16(18).

Simopoulos, A. P. (2008). The importance of the Omega-6/Omega-3 fatty acid ratio in cardiovascular disease and other chronic diseases. Experimental Biology and Medicine, 223(6).

Edwards, R., el al. (1998). Omega-3 polyunsaturated fatty acid levels in the diet and in red blood cell membranes of depressed patients. Journal of Affective Disorders, 48.

Frasure-Smith, N., Lesperance, F., & Pierre, J. (2004). Major Depression is Associated with Lower Omega-3 Fatty Acid Levels in Patients with Recent Acute Coronary Syndromes. Biological Psychiatry, 55.

Jacka, F. N., et al. (2009). Association between magnesium intake and depression and anxiety in community-dwelling adults: the Hordaland Health Study. The Australian and New Zealand Journal of Psychiatry, 43(1).

Walker, A., et al. (2009). Magnesium Supplementation Alleviates Premenstrual Symptoms of Fluid Retention. Journal of Women's Health, 7.

Bottiglieri, T. (2005). Homocysteine and folate metabolism in depression. Progress in Neuro-psychopharmacology and Biological Psychiatry.

Syed, E. U., et al. (2013). Vitamin B12 supplementation in treatment of major depressive disorder: a randomised controlled trial. The Open Neurology Journal.

Owen, A. J. (2005). Low plasma vitamin E levels in major depression: diet or disease? European Journal of Clinical Nutrition, 59.

Lambert, N. M., et al. (2011). Gratitude and depressive symptoms: role of positive reframing and positive emotion. Cognition and Emotion, 26(4).